What Healthcare Professi

The Rite Way t

"Dr. Rite has done a masterful job of describing healing energy principles, and presents in clear and simple language how to prevent chronic illnesses with easy-to-remember rules anyone can follow. His description of the invisible etheric body that surrounds the physical and its relationship to health is not taught in medical schools today but will be soon. His exposure of sugar toxins, contained in most processed foods, is comprehensive and easy to understand and is a major health service to the public."

R. Bieler, O.M.D., Licensed Acupuncturist,
Costa Mesa, CA.

"Having referred numerous patients to Dr. Rite, I'm impressed with the way he educates patients on simple everyday lifestyle practices that will prevent some of the most deadly diseases. Dr. Rite deserves credit for his wellness and longevity concepts that are made easy to understand in the form of 7 simple but powerful rules. His patients are walking testaments to the effectiveness of prevention and healing energy rules as advocated in The Rite Way book."

M. Matos, M.D.,
Long Beach, CA.

"I have witnessed the effectiveness of Dr. Rite's 7 Rules in overcoming premature aging, obesity, diabetes, heart disease, and many gastrointestinal diseases including parasites and tenacious microbial infections with his patients. If you're seeking high levels of wellness and energy and want to become a healthy centenarian, his book is a must read."

T. Le, Licensed Doctor of Chiropractic,
Westminster, CA.

"I have referred many obese patients to Dr. Rite and he is consistently able to coach them into using the 7 Rite Rules to achieve remarkable healthy weight loss. He uses the same techniques as described in The Rite Way book to get patients to overcome bad habits and change their lifestyles for good."

G. Gottshalk, M.D.,
Irvine, CA.

THE RITE WAY TO IMMORTALITY

7 Rite Rules of Wellness, Energy & Longevity

F. Catanza Rite, Ph.D., D.H.H.

authorHOUSE®

AuthorHouse™
1663 Liberty Drive, Suite 200
Bloomington, IN 47403
www.authorhouse.com
Phone: 1-800-839-8640

First published by AuthorHouse 03/11/2009

ISBN: 1-9781-4389-61934

Printed in the United States of America
Bloomington, Indiana

This book is printed on acid-free paper.

Dedication

In memory of my mother, Helen, my father Bruno, and my brother John. All of them would probably be alive today if they knew about the wellness and longevity wisdom contained within this book.

This work is also dedicated to my four children Jeffrey, Laurie, Cathy and Bruce. I am pleased and gratified that they are, by and large, living The Rite Way. They are truly wonderful human beings and I consider myself blessed and fortunate to have them in my life.

Acknowledgment

I must acknowledge the important contributions made by Renee M. Wilmeth in the editing of this work. Her insights and knowledge of wellness and longevity issues made an enormous contribution in adding understanding and clarity to some very challenging health concepts that would have otherwise been very difficult to portray and properly grasp.

Table of Contents

A new perspective on immortality

The reader is asked to consider an extension of bodily life in 3 phases. The 1st phase includes following all of the 7 Rite Rules contained in this work plus adhering to the section on How to Change and Remove Bad Habits. Following these precepts will likely keep you free of disease and in 10 to 20 years keep your mind and body ready to accept new phase 2 therapies. They will come from the sciences of Nutrigenomics and Stem Cell research that includes glyco-protein applications and defective cell replacements. The targeted application of these nutrients will promote full expression of good genes that are known to enhance wellness and energy and keep one free from disease. The nutrients will also have the capacity to suppress genes that are known to have a propensity for causing diseases of debilitation and mortality. Stem cell replacement offers the prospect of replacing all defective cells and may obviate the need for phase 3 below.

Phase 3 applications center around the sciences of Nano-technologies and Artificial Intelligence and we will have the ability to inject intelligent nanobots into our cells. These enhanced intelligent cells could then detect and destroy pathogens, plus cancer cells, and replace defective genes and even regrow human body parts such as new tissue, organs, and limbs. Regrowth of body parts may develop to an extent where an elderly human could reverse their bio age and be re-made to function at the level of a 21 year old. As a reminder, the phase 2 and 3 fantastic developments may only be applicable if you commit to following the 7 Rite Rules contained in Phase I as detailed in this book.

Preface

Many ancient documents tell us about the creation of the human body and the concept of longevity, including the Bible and ancient Eastern and Tibetan documents. The Bible tells us God created the earth in 6 days and rested on the 7th (about 5 billion years to you and me). He created Adam, then Eve from one of Adam's ribs. They propagated the earth. Elders like Noah and Methuselah lived to ripe old ages—900 years by some reports.

Other great stories from ancient Eastern documents tell us that roughly 5 billion years after Earth's creation, God directed a thousand angels to design a physical human body for Souls to use as a vehicle while on Earth. According to ancient documents in Tibet, it took the angels an equivalent of 100,000 earth years to complete the design. Whether the body we inhabit today was created by God from a rib or by angels by cosmic design, we know that it is a complex organic machine. It consists of thousands of separate nerves, bones, muscles, organs, glands, a brain, and other complex subsystems, including a "holy city" (the uterus) where new bodies can be grown, culminating in 60 trillion cells, all designed to work harmoniously within a human body. There are some spiritualists who consider the human body to be the one temple in the universe and that there is nothing holier than this high form; that we are the miracle of miracles—the great inscrutable mystery of God!

The human body was designed so that many of its functions operate automatically, requiring little attention so long as nothing is done to impede its divine wisdom. If properly maintained with the right food, water, energy, exercise, and toxin-free living, the body can last for a very long time. But there's another factor: the spirit.

Whether you believe your body is a temple created by God or a divine vehicle for your karmic Soul, the physical health of your body takes on a much more important meaning. The wisdom of the ages teaches us that as humans we are really spiritual beings with an everlasting Soul temporarily incarnating in many human physical bodies over vast periods of time. The Bible makes reference repeatedly to the teachings of Jesus, the disciples, and other Masters of wisdom, telling us that we are in fact "created in the image of God."

If one accepts the notion, as many ageless writings suggest, that some of the smallest units of matter—sub-atomic particles and atoms—have a consciousness, then the logic of molecular and cellular consciousness follows because they are made up of sub-atomic particles and atoms. With this relationship in mind it is reasonable to assume that our cells, all 60 trillion of them, hold a consciousness of a power greater than themselves and for them that power is what they are literally living inside... a human body. To these small entities, living within our bodies, isn't it reasonable to expect their consciousness to regard us humans, the body they are living within, as God?

Molecules, the Body, and the Universe

If you think of the body as a divine entity, it explains a larger divine relationship between humans and the cosmos all the way up the cosmic chain (and down it as well) showing our place in regard to God's universal body, the world, and even the universe. Thinking cosmically as well as spiritually about the concept "as below so above," we can view our place on the planet Earth as living upon an electron within an atom called the solar system. From a cosmic perspective, our solar system is but one of many atoms within a constellation. Constellations could be equivalent to molecules within a galaxy cell of a larger being and humans, living in this cell, within the atom of our solar system on the electron Earth, could be equivalent to sub-atomic particles within the atom.

If we view our solar system as an atom and part of a cosmic molecular structure made up of myriad other solar systems, cosmically they are only molecules making up parts of a cell. But a cell of what? Maybe a cell of God's body called the "Milky Way Galaxy"? Or maybe something bigger? When you start to think about this idea, you start to get a sense of man and the possible relationship to the image of God—God as the universe within which humans are breathing, eating, moving, and living. You also start to get a glimpse of the expansiveness and awesome exquisiteness of man and his relationship to God as the universe.

Here's another way to look at it. If we use the logic that many constellations (molecules) are needed to make up just one cell (a galaxy), then it follows we can reasonably predict how many galaxies there probably are in the universe. Now, think about that in relationship to the human body. Since we know there are about 60 trillion cells in the human body, the law of correspondence tells us that this is about how many cells there are in the universe—or the whole body of God—since we're made in His image. It nearly staggers the imagination to try and comprehend the size of 60 trillion galaxies and the number of solar systems and planets that actually make up the universe. And we live in it, within one of His cells, a galaxy called the Milky Way, within a molecular constellation called Sirius, within an atom called the solar system, and on this tiny electron speck of a planet called Earth, we as sub-atomic particles called human beings eat, sleep, move, and live. (If you follow string theory, then you know that it postulates that there are many universes and that some string theorists claim that the number of universes could be limitless. But we're not going to go into that here.)

It is nearly impossible, with the limitations of the human mind and limitations of what we can see with telescopes and hear with radio astronomy, to describe what an organ, let alone a cell, might look like within the body of God. But it is reasonable to believe that they may look like the organs and cells inside a human body based on the law of correspondence and the law of "as below so above."

It is humbling to realize that we as sub-atomic particles have bodies that live for less than a flash of time in the universe—the cosmic body of God. And if we look at the current universal physical body to be about 15 billion years old and measure it against a typical human body, currently living about 75 years, one can get a sense of just how short human physical bodies live, cosmically speaking. It's the equivalent of sub-atomic particles flashing in and out of existence within the human body in your daily existence.

The Real Possibility of Immortality

So what does all this mean in relation to my 7 Rite Rules? I wrote this book in the hope that it may prove useful to all open-minded seekers of truth who want to create good karma while in their present bodies by keeping them healthy. It is also directed to all those who view their bodies as a temple and desire to optimize their life span, placing them on the path to a vibrant and healthy centenarian age and beyond. Some Masters of wisdom claim that we are entering an age of increased cosmic ray energies, which may offer longer life spans to many people. It could become a reality that many more will live to be 100 years and beyond—and maybe eventually to the age of Methuselah of 900+ years. At the very least, the age of an everlasting physical body is rapidly becoming more possible if the Soul chooses to keep one, and only one, body.

Many people (those under 35, in particular) have little desire to live more than 100 years. Their image of a centenarian is one of a lifestyle of sickliness and decrepitness, dependent on others for survival. Many believe they have little or no control over how long they will live, that their genetics predetermine their life span, and their lifestyle has little to do with their level of wellness and longevity.

This work aims to dispel many of these notions and to provide a logical program of systemic rules for living not only a long life, but an active and healthy one. Each person can play a role in upgrading their personal health and that of their friends, families, and the general population. It also is intended to raise the level of consciousness beyond the current physical mantra of "more of every material thing is good" and to help readers realize that true wellness is not just a question of living a healthier, longer life. I hope to make readers think about what the positive impact may be from a disease-free life and its effects on the spiritual real self... the Soul.

In this book, I recognize that at least 80 percent of the population exhibits a profile of over-consumption of adulterated foods, recreational drugs (including caffeine and alcohol), prescription drugs, over-the-counter medications, and other indulgences. Many have built up a lifetime of bad habits, feeding on heavy consumption of processed foods, sodas, caffeine, alcohol, and prescription medications, all supported by a sedentary lifestyle and reinforced by media advertising. If a high percentage of the majority were to change and follow my prescribed wellness and longevity principles, our population's health would measurably improve and national health care costs would drop dramatically. And, if only a small percentage can be persuaded to change, I would consider it sufficient justification for the effort put forth to create and publish this book. Think of it in terms of how valuable it would be if you could influence a small number of sub-atomic particles within your body to behave in a beneficial way to support the orderliness of your cells, molecules, and organs. And think about the quote "we are all connected" and how it relates to supporting the orderliness of the planet and its probable relationship to the wellness of the universe.

Ultimately, this work will carry its message to the hearts and minds of those currently on the wellness path and to those ready to make lifestyle changes. All that can be asked of the reader of this work is an open-mindedness and willingness to consider the views put forth, and that honesty and sincerity of thought will lead to a rejection of the false and an appreciation of the true causes of disease.

Terms Used in the Text

The term "Master" is used often throughout this work and generally refers to those human beings who are masterful teachers and have developed an extraordinary level of consciousness and desire to serve humanity. Their elevated level of consciousness has been characterized as the difference between that of an intelligent human being compared to one of a chimpanzee. It is said that virtually all humans have the potential to become a Master if they choose to be initiated and follow certain precepts that will raise their consciousness to levels of high enlightenment. Masters are also known to meditate several hours a day and generally advocate harmlessness, self-realization, and service to humanity. Examples of Masters through the ages up to the present include Moses, Buddha, Krishna, St. Francis, Loa Tse, Socrates, Plato, Christ, Muhammad, Sawan Singhji, Yogananda, Djwhal Khul, Ching Hai, and others. Several of these Masters are referenced throughout this work regarding their thoughts on the Soul, etheric body, physical body, karma, and a variety of health and spiritual issues.

Although this work is directed to those seeking reliable information that can be acted upon to promote wellness, energy, and longevity, it is also intended for the health professionals and universities to ponder on the appropriateness of establishing research programs to support, with factual data and scientific methods, the existence of the Soul. I also hope that it will help lead to the recognition of the etheric and other unseen energy bodies referenced in this work.

Introduction

Living the Rite Way and Being "Drop-Dead Healthy"

Up until the age of 35 I ate the Standard American Diet, what I call the SAD diet, one filled with burgers, fries, sodas, donuts, coffee, chips, and pizza, all the while paying little attention to proper rest, exercise, and toxins. Like many Americans, I thought my lifestyle was good. In fact, I had a smug and positive attitude that my lifestyle was in fact healthy. I suppose that some would have characterized me as having an air of invincibility until my annual physical uncovered signs of serious cardiovascular problems. I did some intensive research on heart illnesses and began looking into patterns of disease among my relatives and friends.

Nearly all of my relatives and several of my close friends died unhealthy, miserably, and painfully from some form of chronic disease. My Grandmother Bertha, who was an immigrant from Russia, dropped dead unhealthy at the age of 42 from kidney disease, followed by my Grandfather Charles, an immigrant from Lithuania, who dropped dead painfully from heart disease at 57. My Grandmother Catherine, an immigrant from Italy, died unhealthy at the age of 67 from stomach cancer, followed by my father Bruno, who died a bedridden, painful death at the age of 56 from colon cancer. His sister, my Aunt Peggy, died miserably from diabetes at the age of 61, and her husband Gene had a stroke and lived several unhappy and frustrating years as an invalid until he dropped dead unhealthy at the age of 66 from another stroke. My Dad's brother, my Uncle Joe, died extremely sick and miserable at the age of 74 from prostate cancer after being bedridden for nearly a year. My mother Helen outlived them all, but her last ten years were filled with debilitating events ranging from a heart attack to several strokes. She dropped dead unhealthy from a final heart attack at the age of 83.

I know you're thinking "what a family history!" I'll spare you the details regarding several of my friends and neighbors who also dropped dead unhealthy and prematurely from chronic illnesses. One common thread? Virtually all of the described friends and relatives were either grossly overweight and/or morbidly obese.

The keynote of this book is to teach people how to live long and vibrantly and prevent illnesses by following the 7 Rite Rules of Energy, Wellness, and Longevity. Why do I call it "drop-dead healthy"? Have you ever heard a beautiful woman described as "drop-dead gorgeous"? It's a great image, right? So is "drop-dead healthy." It should describe how you will look and feel if you follow the 7 Rite Rules. Dying drop-dead healthy instills an image of possibilities for a disease-free life where one in fact can "drop-dead healthy" if one chooses to do so.

The shared experience with my relatives in some ways reflects just how poor America's health picture is, with nearly 70 percent of people being overweight. For example, obesity correlates high with increased risk for cardiovascular disease, cancer, diabetes, strokes, hypertension, excess fatigue, sleep apnea, kidney disorders, and urinary incontinence. In simple terms, these illnesses indicate a lifestyle of over-consumption (excess energy input), low levels of hydration, poor rest, and physical inactivity. If lifestyle changes are not made to correct for the above conditions it is probable that one or more of those diseases will manifest. Those afflicted will likely experience a life filled with fatigue, and assisted care requirements leading to morbid and pain-filled, premature death—that is, dropping dead unhealthy!

After I recognized my own unhealthy patterns, that realization planted the seeds for developing a consciousness of disease prevention. It also inspired me to become a holistic doctor. As I built my practice and continued my research, I found myself developing an evangelistic fervor to spread the word about prevention and tell anyone who would listen about how to "prevent disease and reclaim your health." I, myself, learned to live The Rite Way. You can too!

Calendar Age vs. Biological Age

When I became a practicing holistic doctor I began to measure nearly every anti-aging patient's biological age based on the following bio-markers: muscle mass, body fat, body hydration, hand and body strength, dexterity, skin elasticity, and phase angle, plus over a dozen heart markers, some of which included cholesterol, low density lipids, high density lipids, blood pressure, triglycerides, C-reactive protein, homocysteine, and several other fat markers.

At my calendar age of 54 I had a biological age of 47; today at age 68 my biological age is 41, and many of my patients who have learned to live The Rite Way have had similar results. In other words, the older they are chronologically, the younger they are getting biologically! As strange as it may seem, the ability to reverse biological age is a fact. My patients and I have learned how to do it by following the 7 Rite Rules.

I've included details on how to measure and correlate each bio-marker to the calendar and biological age in the appendix. As will be shown in several of the following chapters, body composition measurements regarding muscle, fat, and water percentages are among the most reliable and telling markers for accurately measuring biological age. As of this writing, at calendar age 68, my body is composed of 13% fat, and 87% lean tissue and water. In addition to body composition, phase angle has also gained prominence as a significant bio-marker. In essence, this marker measures the amount of hydration within and outside the cell membranes. My phase angle measured 9.5, and a typical 68-year-old male measures about 6.0. A 9.5 phase angle is seldom found among those over 40 years old. History of illness is a bio-marker that accounts for how many times an illness has occurred over the past three years. This marker measures the effectiveness of the immune system and fortunately, due to living The Rite Way, I have not had any bouts of illness for the past 17 years. These numbers coupled with other bio-markers compute to a 41 year biological age. Achieving this bio-number meant following all of the 7 Rite Rules.

I recommend measuring the bio-markers at the start of an anti-aging program, but due to the cost (approximately $900) some patients decide to follow the program without doing the objective measurements. Patients in general who subjectively rate their condition after the clinical anti-aging experience claim new-found energies and freedom from illnesses, and everyone remarks on looking and feeling younger after about three to four months on The 7 Rite Rules Program. So, objective measurements are available, but if you decide to do the program without them you can expect to experience noticeable improvements over a 3–4 month period by following The 7 Rite Rules.

Living a Long Healthy Life The Rite Way

Beth, at 103 years old, is as careful about her appearance as she is about the food she buys fresh every day for her meals. Every morning on her way out the door, she stops by the mirror in the hall to run a brush through her thick hair and dab on her favorite lipstick. Sammy, her ancient beagle-terrier, does a little dance, tail wagging, as Beth fetches the leash, and the two of them set out on their four-block trek to the market.

No sad picture of advanced age, Beth lives independently, enjoying visits with friends and family. Her mind is sharp enough to beat her great-nephew at cards and she loves listening to books on tape while Sammy naps at her feet. She also enjoys having her great-grandchildren over for dinner, giving her the opportunity to share their company and to educate them on the importance of living The Rite Way, letting orderly energies from wholesome food, water, and air into their bodies. She gets a great deal of satisfaction passing on what she learned as a registered nurse while working with several Eastern medical doctors. She understands, having lived a long, healthy life The Rite Way, that all disease is related to energy as it passes through the body in either excess or deficiency.

Beth has never taken medications, and has always had high levels of energy. Astonishingly, she cannot remember a single day of illness in her entire adult life, even though both her parents died at age 69 from cancer, and all four grandparents succumbed to either heart disease or stroke, none living beyond the age of 74.

Beth does not owe her longevity and vitality to either genetics or luck. She earned it by virtue of her lifestyle. In fact, her lifestyle is a near-perfect mirror of The 7 Rite Rules of Wellness, Energy, and Longevity, optimizing biological age and living a disease-free, long, energetic life. Beth lived her life The Rite Way according to the rules. You can too!

You Can Learn to Make The Rite Choices

As thinking adults we have choices regarding aging. One can follow the rules of wellness, energy, and longevity and likely live far beyond today's predicted life span, even become a centenarian. However, one can live a lifestyle of undisciplined indulgence and likely incur painful and morbid diseases and drop dead unhealthy at an average age of 74 years.

There are some health practitioners who claim that all of the sicknesses related to aging should be compressed into the last few years of life. Some doctors think it's desirable to achieve this illness state later in life. This concept is unacceptable to me. It doesn't make sense that if the body was not designed to be filled with illnesses at any period of one's life, it would be suited to being ill during the later stages of life.

As stated repeatedly in this work, one of the major principles from which The Rite Rules flow is based on the ancient fact that the human body was designed by a divine intelligence. This intelligence results in an innate bodily wisdom providing perfect operation insofar as no impediments block this inscrutable wisdom.

Our responsibility as humans is to live The Rite Way to ensure that nothing impedes this wonderful bodily wisdom while we, as Souls, are living in this miraculous bodily vehicle, allowing us to enjoy this life on earth.

The Connection to Wellness and Longevity

Most people have not made the connection that negative lifestyle habits adversely affect wellness and longevity. Many hold the view that their genetics dominate health status and that lifestyle has little influence. This denial is one reason the health profile of Americans continues to decline.

Physically we are a people suffering from many morbid diseases as we age. The majority of Americans are sedentary couch potatoes addicted to watching more than six hours of television per day. Many are compulsive overeaters, and consume foods at the highest rate per capita of any nation. We spend more than 1.5 trillion dollars per year on so-called health care, which in fact should be termed "sickness care." Most people connect health insurance to a healthy life. Very few people think in terms of prevention of illness, but instead believe that they can live any way they desire and their doctors, covered by their health insurance, will cure them of most ills.

A Nation of Medicine Chest Addicts

We are a nation of medicine chest addicts. Whether over the counter or prescription, the general belief is that the answer to all illness rests in finding the right drug to cover up the pain and/or symptoms of arthritis, asthma, allergies, fatigue, indigestion, and obesity. The thought of preventing these chronic diseases through proper lifestyles—early on before it's too late—is not part of the general population's mindset. We are generally overdosed with advertising and overly influenced by processed foods, pharmaceuticals, insurance, and medical industry propaganda, so much so that it has created a system of spreading large-scale misunderstandings and misinformation. As a consequence, it is reasonable to predict that chronic illnesses will accelerate and the cost of "sickness care" will continue to escalate.

We are in many respects victims of our own prosperity, gorging and choking on the effects of over-consumption. We tend to view any abstinence or restriction on lifestyle as an infringement on satisfaction and happiness. I often hear "These satisfactions help me live a full life." When I suggest the patient cut back or eliminate certain kinds of processed foods or alcoholic drinks, I often hear "what's the sense of living a longer life if I can't enjoy the food and drink that tastes good and makes me feel good?" Here's another one: "I'd rather be dead than to have to give up that food." I hear that when I suggest giving up coffee, alcohol, processed foods, and sugar. In most situations these recommendations are directed to those who are suffering from serious chronic problems such as heart disease, obesity, hypertension, or diabetes. But, many people are literally slaves to their sense of taste, and the thought of being free from a particular compulsion is not part of their consciousness. For the most part they can generally be described as being in a state of denial with an inability for recognizing any type of problem or consequence created by their behavior.

Health Information Overload

The promise to humanity of a future with golden health and extended life has turned out to be seemingly empty. Degenerative diseases—heart attacks, strokes, cancer, arthritis, obesity, diabetes, hypertension, ulcers, chronic fatigue, irritable bowel syndrome, and the rest—have replaced the infectious diseases of 100 years ago as the major enemies of life and destroyers of its quality. There are many theories and lots of conflicting information on what may be best for the health and longevity of individuals in our society. However, in the broad scope of health, there is relatively little accurate information we can rely on.

"Errors and untruths run down an incline plane, but truths have to climb a mountain."

—H. Blavatsky

Today there are numerous diet, exercise, and lifestyle systems that promise longevity, fat loss, increased energy, and freedom from disease. Major book stores stock hundreds of titles on personal health and wellness and related self-improvement matters. Various universities and medical schools publish dozens of different health advisory letters. Radio and television programs in every part of the U.S. devote time to health-related issues, and almost every major newspaper has a health section of some sort. One is nearly overwhelmed with the avalanche of magazines entirely devoted to health issues, and the health-related articles touted on the covers of most other women's and men's magazines.

Beyond the print, radio, and television media there are hundreds of seminars and meetings offered annually, monthly, and weekly by local health food stores, drug companies, and nutritional product manufacturers. Then there is the Internet, with thousands of web sites devoted to health information, diseases, conditions, symptoms, patients, support, and recommendations for those seeking specific answers to a wide variety of wellness and illness concerns.

Garbage In, Garbage Out

While all of these sources look like good news for those interested in obtaining health information, it also presents a challenge regarding misinformation, information overload, and resulting confusion on the part of the general public. Moreover, there is a great deal of conflicting data regarding what is truly good and what is bad for health. Some would say that there are those who are intentionally misleading the public in order to push their products and services.

Who Can Be Trusted for Accurate Health Information?

As a reader, you should always consider the source. For example, the large processed food manufacturers, meat producers, dairy industries, vitamin product manufacturers, and pharmaceutical companies all have a vested interest in helping you, the consumer, believe that consuming their products is healthy. From an early age, we learn about eating right using the four food groups, and then we learn that vitamin supplements and other medicines are necessary to maintain health or overcome illness, even though many educated adults today know or suspect that these accepted practices can't be blindly trusted. While there is a fair amount of dispute over the pros and cons of animal products, vitamins, and pharmaceuticals, there is little doubt in scientific circles regarding the long-term negative health effects of the majority of processed foods. We all have concerns about a vast array of chemical ingredients, harmful processing, packaging, and storage techniques mostly used to help the product be more appealing to taste, appearance, and a longer shelf life.

It is not that food firms are trying to produce bad food. It is more a matter of them not trying to produce good food. They are trying to produce profits, and they have learned that in order to expand their markets and profits, they must sweeten their products, add humectants, add color dyes, add preservatives, add flavor chemicals, and so on. When flavors, colors, and preservatives are synthesized with the food, manufacturers are freed from dealing with the cost and concerns of real foods found in the produce section of supermarkets.

In an overall strategic sense, processed food manufacturers are attempting to design foods to appeal to consumers—particularly children—that will meet real or imagined wants and needs. Whether these foods are ultimately healthy or harmful is not their major concern. (Chapter 7 examines the specifics of harmful additives, processing, animal products, and pharmaceutical toxins.)

In many respects, the lack of integrity regarding health information can be viewed as a collective world tragedy with an intellectual dishonesty that rivals even the most treacherous of propaganda machines. The deliberate untruths and misleading information spread by many politically motivated and commercially inspired companies can be viewed as negative forces thriving on disease, and on profits from their products that cause or contribute to a vast array of illnesses. The erroneous health ideas that are propagated enslave people mentally and emotionally every bit as much as some national institutions have enslaved people physically. The powerful alliance of some government agencies, drug companies, food manufacturers, supplement manufacturers, and meat, dairy, and alcohol industries should be of concern to all of you. They often monopolize all paths of information and education by initiating or supporting research, and publishing fabricated findings to support their self-serving interests.

The general public is often left bewildered and confused with no clear answers as to what path to follow for achieving freedom from disease and lasting health and wellness. As a result, the majority of the public literally poison their bodies with toxins every day, contributing to their ill health and the escalating costs associated with overall health care.

Can You Accept the Truth?

In dealing with the issues surrounding information on physical wellness, it is necessary to know what assumptions are held by certain sources when they make claims for what is good or bad for the human body. In examining the motives and perceived agendas of most of the institutions mentioned above, it is clear that when they speak it is from a self-serving motive. This can also be the case when an individual is putting forth a position on a product or a service in which he or she may have a vested interest. Therefore, it seems to me it is incumbent upon the producer of health information to present or reveal any and all ties to companies, products, and/or services that may prejudice their viewpoints.

The Truth? The Body Has a Built-in Wisdom

You don't have to spend a lifetime educating yourself about all aspects of health in order to live a healthy life. All you need is the right information to keep your body as healthy as possible. You need The 7 Rite Rules—a plan that embodies seven principles designed to cover all the basics that you need to know for maximizing health and longevity. The plan and principles are based on natural laws and truths supported by many health researchers, practitioners, and Masters of ageless wisdom.

In this work I advocate no products or services... only unbiased rules known to prevent disease, increase molecular energy, and promote longevity.

I am not sure anyone can be entirely unbiased when imparting health information, so with that point in mind I believe a statement of philosophy and assumptions is in order before I present my prescription for wellness, energy, and longevity, and let the reader judge my plan accordingly.

Based on considerable research and practical experience over a 30-year period, I have come to embrace and synthesize much of the ancient wisdom of Eastern Masters, Greek philosophers, Hebrew, Christian, and modern Masters of wisdom in their expressed universal healing truths, together with other health practitioners and my practical findings. The essentials are worth repeating and are as follows: The wisdom contained within the human body is enormous and powerful, and it is in essence the same wisdom and power that stems from the divine body of intelligence that designed and created the universe and all of us within in it. This body wisdom can also be viewed as the Soul within the body, and to the extent that the mind and body will comply with the desires of the Soul, the body actually will not require much attention.

This bodily wisdom and intelligence dwarfs the power of any one human doctor or healer. Beyond accidents and initial acute emergency treatment from medical doctors, the body wisdom and intelligence are the only forces that can restore health and functional integrity. But, as shown in this work, the major emphasis on preserving human health should be on preventing illnesses through proper lifestyle practices. It is on this point of prevention that the 7 Rite Rules of Wellness, Energy, and Longevity are directed. These rules embody the precepts of ancient wisdom documents, many classical Masters, and modern-day health practitioners.

In relating these principles I can assure the reader that there is no hidden agenda that might prejudice or slant the presentation of truths that I hold to be virtually inscrutable and sacred. The underlying premise, which is repeated often in this work, is that everyone's level of health lies in the ability to have the mind, body, and emotions disciplined sufficiently to "dance to the rhythm of the Soul" by allowing this innate wisdom to flourish and flow unimpeded by following the natural rhythm embodied in the principles of Rite eating, drinking, resting, energizing, exercising, believing, and toxin-free living. It is interesting to note that none of these practices require undue attention to the body; it is primarily a matter of allowing the body, a marvelous automaton, to function perfectly until the Soul decides it is time to leave.

An Easy Way to Remember The 7 Rite Rules of Wellness

Initially, I advocated five rules to achieve wellness and longevity. However, in my lectures and presentations, it became clear to me that the diet principle was too lengthy with the inclusion of foods, liquids, and toxins, so I added separate rules to cover the latter two. Additionally, several patients gave me the idea of using my professional name, so they became The 7 Rite Rules of **D**iet, **R**est, **R**ays, **I**mbibement, **T**oxin-free Living, **E**xercise, and **S**oulfulness.

As I've written and polished this book, I've given considerable thought as to how the general public can conveniently remember these truths and employ them on a daily basis when there is so much confusion regarding health information out there today. The D-R-R-I-T-E-S acronym is intended as a simple and effective method for remembering what is needed through Rite Diet, Rite Rest, Rite Rays, Rite Imbibement, Rite Toxin-free Living, Rite Exercise, and Rite Soulfulness. (The Rite Imbibement Rule replaces liquids, and the Rite Toxin-free Living Rule expands on the toxin principle originally included in the Diet Rule.)

In summary, the D-R-R-I-T-E-S rules are as follows:

Rite **D**iet: why, what kind, and how much food to eat.
Rite **R**est: why, when, and how much rest is needed.
Rite **R**ays: why, what kind, and how much unseen energies are needed.
Rite **I**mbibement: why, what kind, and how much water is needed.
Rite **T**oxin-free Living: why and what kinds of products cause disease.
Rite **E**xercise: why, what kind, how, and how much exercise is needed.
Rite **S**oulfulness: why and how emotions, body, and mind are controlled.

Beyond the logic of the D-R-R-I-T-E-S acronym for remembering the rules, you can also view their meaningfulness as a balanced flow of energy outputs from organized energy inputs as related to four states of matter in solid, liquid, gas, and etheric form. Their connection along with the important underlying relationship to Toxin-free Living and Soulfulness works in a system of layers:

> **Top Layer:** Energy Outputs—Rite Rest, Rite Exercise
> **Middle Layer:** Energy Inputs—Solids (Rite Eating), Liquids (Rite Drinking), Gasses and Etheric (Rite Breathing and Rite Rays)
> **Foundation Layer:** Rite Toxin-free Living
> **Rite Soulfulness:** a rhythmic and balanced flow of organized energy within and between the physical, emotional, mental, and spiritual bodies

Each of The 7 Rite Rules are described and explained in detail in separate chapters. I have presented this plan to hundreds of patients and nearly all of them have benefited substantially from a physical health standpoint. Whether they will live longer than they otherwise would have remains to be seen and may be open to question. However, the physical health benefits, including significant increases in energy and a vibrant zest for life, freedom from pain, and a general sense of well-being and fitness, cannot be denied by the majority of those employing these principles.

The rules are primarily delineated to serve as a lifestyle guide for preventing chronic health problems. However, from a patient's standpoint, for those having developed one or more chronic illnesses, these rules possibly could also serve to help overcome many chronic disorders.

The Rules Are Simple; Adherence Is a Challenge

This prescription, simple as it is, doesn't work for everyone due primarily to patient compliance. The problem of patient compliance is dealt with in depth in Chapter 2, "The Rite Way to Change for Life." But for any program to be successful, you have to know what ought to be done to achieve and maintain health and then implement it. There are many forces working to impede good intentions, but I encourage you to know that there are proven technologies to help facilitate and bring about prescribed changes. Once you understand the change process and the importance of each stage, you'll have a different perspective on implementing successful, long-term change.

The primary forces that impede health compliance with the majority of people today have to do with the formation of unhealthy habits. Emotions are in fact at the base of most unhealthy habit formations, and the underlying problem with emotional domination has to do with low levels of consciousness and the lack of mental control. There is, in essence, a disconnection with the Soul.

In this book, I work from the fundamental idea that the primary, underlying root of most disease is related to the excess or deficiency of energy as it pours through the body centers. I bring this up now because these energy flows do have a direct physical relation to the body. I also bring it up because in explaining these principles throughout the book, you may get a spiritual perspective and begin to feel this approach is a little too esoteric for you. Before you begin to look elsewhere for answers, I encourage you to focus on the very real steps in this book that you can take to physically improve your body and open your mind to some other concepts that may affect your health; concepts that your traditional Western doctor may not necessarily believe in.

The reader can be assured, from a practical standpoint, that they will substantially benefit from this book even if they choose not to embrace the existence of higher spiritual planes. Having said that, I believe that those who do choose to read The Rite Soulfulness chapter with an open mind will find a perspective developing that can lead to creating a lasting and healthy change for this life.

Creating a Lasting, Healthy Change

In creating a lasting, healthy change for this life, I ask the reader to ponder the effects on a subsequent body when the Soul is free from all past and present negative predilections. The concept of The Rite Way to Immortality takes on an eternal perspective that includes the effects on past, present, and future physical bodies for our Souls. It means that living The Rite Way in this life offers the possibility for immortality in the present body, and certainly the everlasting immortal Soul will benefit with a new body in the event the present body becomes no longer useful for one's Soul.

In the here and now of the present life, where the prospects of physical immortality may seem too remote to even consider, the reader is asked to follow The 7 Rite Rules in this work and think in terms of staying well in mind and body for the next 15 to 25 years. This time view is suggested as a promising period to be alive with sound mind and body in order to take advantage of new cosmic energies and new medical developments. Several prominent anti-aging and longevity researchers have repeatedly claimed that the prospects for physical immortality are imminent and the promise may be just a few decades away.

As an example, according to Kurzweil and Dr. Grossman in their book Fantastic Voyage, "we are in the early stages of multiple profound revolutions spawned by the intersection of biology, information science, and nano technology. With the decoding of the human genome, new powerful drugs designed for precise missions without side effects, regrowing new cells, tissues, and organs, reversing the aging process, gene therapy, and nanorobots placed in our bodies the size of blood cells to enhance every aspect of our lives are transformations some of which are available today."

They and others in anti-aging research point out the way to something humans have only dreamed about until now—the promise of living forever.

The Prevention Matrix

The primary purpose for following The 7 Rite Rules is to prevent chronic illnesses. When one does contract a chronic illness it is most likely due to a violation of one or more of the rules. The rules are described in separate chapters with great detail as to why each is important in preventing chronic illnesses. The matrix of chronic illnesses outlined in this section helps clarify the potential relationship of each principle to specific chronic illnesses.

Ben Franklin's adage "an ounce of prevention is worth a pound of cure" has particular significance regarding health matters. In some respects it actually represents an understated condition of the real difference between the cost and effort required to prevent an illness versus the cost and effort to cure an illness. Preventing illnesses such as heart disease, cancer, and strokes, which are the three leading causes of death in America, can show dramatic cost benefits. The cost of prevention to cost of cure can far exceed the ounce-to-pound ratio when the following examples are examined: An individual with heart disease requiring surgery for a heart bypass can easily incur costs exceeding $50,000 just for doctor and hospital expenses. Cancer patients commonly incur costs of several hundred thousand dollars for various kinds of surgery, radiation, and chemotherapy treatments. Stroke victims regularly run up rehabilitation therapy costs well above $100,000. In all of these examples, the loss of wages and reduced quality of life should also be factored into the cost of cure.

The interesting aspect regarding the cost of prevention versus the cost of cure is that in the majority of prevention examples there are virtually no added costs. In fact there are often savings attached to not indulging in actions that violate the rules. This is the case particularly with those rules showing major links to specific diseases like cancer, cardiovascular disease, and strokes.

When examining the list of chronic illnesses shown in the matrix it is clear that proper energy inputs from solid foods, liquids, air, and etheric energies are major factor's in preventing chronic illnesses. The proper processing of these energies in the form of rest, attitude, exercise, and avoidance of toxins are also translated into rules that could have a major impact on prevention of chronic diseases. Those rules deemed to have a major impact are designated with an "M." Those noted with a "C" are classified as likely to contribute to an impact, and rules that may play a role are represented with a lowercase "m."

In order to help get a sense for applying this matrix to real-life situations, a review of a common illness known as "chronic fatigue" is used as an example. Looking across the principle columns, an "M" is located in all seven columns under Diet, Rest, Rays, Imbibe, Toxin-free Lifestyle, Exercise, and Soulfulness.

Translated, this means that a deficiency or imbalance in applying any one of these rules could be a major cause of a "chronic fatigue" condition. (With Toxin-free Lifestyle, the "M" would not represent a deficiency but rather an overdose of toxins as having a major impact.)

It should be understood that multiple rules are at work in preventing nearly every illness, and that in order to prevent the majority of illnesses, adherence to The 7 Rite Rules is advocated.

Prevention is the major theme of this work, but the dynamics of curing disease is another matter and the prevention matrix is not as useful. The curing of diseases can be a time-consuming and costly endeavor involving a whole set of different and often complex dynamics. It offers many opportunities for mischief and errors and when in combination with health insurance coverage, it presents a primary reason for why health care costs are growing at an annual rate of over 10 percent in the USA.

It should be obvious to all that much more emphasis should be placed on the importance of prevention, and this is the theme the reader will find threading its way throughout much of this work.

In reviewing the following matrix it should be clear that the vast majority of diseases are preventable or improvable by any one of The 7 Rite Rules or combinations thereof. In other words, each one is just as important as the others in playing a major role in preventing most diseases. Therefore, the reader should give each rule equal time and study to ensure that they are understood, and particular attention should be given to how they are going to be incorporated into their lifestyle.

The overwhelming number of M designations in the matrix means that the vast majority of illnesses will virtually be prevented when all of the rules are incorporated into one's lifestyle. As preposterous as this may seem to many people, I can attest that it has worked for me and for my patients who are known to have followed the rules.

Toxins can include parasites, bacteria, yeast, viruses, heavy metals, pesticides, preservatives, humectants, fillers, taste enhancers, added hormones, antibiotics, fats, drugs, sugars, and so on. (Although cures are not the subject of this matrix, in many cases some type of specific toxin removal therapy will be required in order to correct most chronic conditions. In addition, most chronic problems require a thorough understanding of the patient's symptoms and lifestyle in order for a cure to be effective on a long-term basis.)

For many conditions, testing for toxins is appropriate and could include hair, urine, saliva, blood, and/or stool analysis to determine levels of toxicity, pathogens, and nutritional deficiencies. Therefore, the specific remedies for overcoming particular diseases can be complex and can make for the subject of an entire book. On the other hand, it could be that a change of lifestyle, employing all of the Rite Rules, could serve to overcome many chronic illnesses and this issue is dealt with in great detail in Chapter 2.

The curing of chronic diseases offers many opportunities for creating additional problems stemming from the misuse of drugs, herbs, vitamins, minerals, and other modalities including unnecessary hospital stays and operations.

The curing process should include informing the doctor that you are interested in more than treating symptoms. You should want to know what will be done to identify the most likely cause, what should be done to remove the cause, and what kinds of risks there are for causing harm in the curing process.

Heart disease, cancer, and strokes are the major diseases causing the bulk of the health insurance premium increases; they are also diseases you can reasonably expect to prevent while living The Rite Way. Huge savings can be created over a lifetime of living The Rite Way by simply converting from comprehensive healthcare insurance, which typically costs $5,000 annually, to catastrophic healthcare insurance, which typically costs $600 annually. If you're self-employed, converting to catastrophic coverage will save you thousands of dollars annually; if you are an employee, you should ask to be converted to catastrophic and have your employer place the difference in a personal health savings account. If your employer needs more information on this alternative, they can e-mail me at the address shown in the Appendix.

Prevention is where the emphasis should be placed in order to have a true "national health care system" as opposed to what is currently a "sickness care system." In the future, I believe all conscientious doctors will feel the need to teach and coach their patients on the lifestyles deemed favorable to prevent chronic illnesses.

Simply curing a chronic disease will not be considered satisfactory unless it is accompanied by information that will educate the patient on what must be done to prevent the disease from re-occurring. Harsh as it may seem, treatment without the teaching prevention effort should be considered as a major disservice and disqualify the practitioner from being referred to as doctor who can effectively help patients cure and prevent further chronic disease of the same order.

Illness Prevention Health Matrix

7 Principles of Wellness & Longevity Related to Prevention of Chronic Illnesses

M=major impact C=likely to contribute m=may have an impact

Chronic Illness	*Diet*	*Rest*	*Rays*	*Imbibe*	*Toxin -free**	*Exercise*	*Soul-fulness*
Aids	M	M	M	M	M	C	M
Alzheimers	M	M	M	M	M	M	M
Allergies	M	M	M	M	M	M	M
Arteriosclerosis	M	M	M	M	M	M	M
Atherosclerosis	M	M	M	M	M	M	M
Arthritis (osteo)	M	M	M	M	M	M	M
Arthritis (rheumatoid)	M	M	M	M	M	M	M
Asthma	M	M	M	M	M	M	M
Bone Spurs	M	M	M	M	M	M	M
Bronchitis	M	M	M	M	M	M	M
Bursitis	M	M	M	M	M	M	M
Cancer	M	M	M	M	M	M	M
Chronic Fat gue	M	M	M	M	M	M	M
Colds (repetitive)	M	M	M	M	M	M	M
Colitis	M	M	M	M	M	M	M
Constipation	M	M	m	M	M	M	M
Crohn's Disease	M	M	M	M	M	M	M
Depression	M	M	M	M	M	M	M
Diabetes	M	M	M	M	M	M	M
Diarrhea	M	M	m	M	M	M	M
Emphysema	M	M	M	M	M	M	M
Fibromyalgia	M	M	M	M	M	M	M
Gallstones	M	M	m	M	M	M	M
Gastritis	M	M	M	M	M	M	M
Gout	M	M	m	M	M	M	M
Graves Disease	M	M	M	M	M	M	M
Headaches	M	M	M	M	M	M	M
Heart Disease	M	M	M	M	M	M	M

Chronic Illness	*Diet*	*Rest*	*Rays*	*Imbibe*	*Toxin -free**	*Exercise*	*Soul-fulness*
Hemorrhoids	M	M	m	M	M	M	M
Hypertension	M	M	M	M	M	M	M
Hypoglycemia	M	M	M	M	M	M	M
Hypothyroidism	M	M	M	M	M	M	M
Kidney Disorders	M	M	M	M	M	M	M
Liver Disease	M	M	M	M	M	M	M
Lupus	M	M	M	M	M	M	M
Meningitis	M	M	M	M	M	M	M
Mononucleosis	M	M	M	M	M	M	M
Multiple Sclerosis	M	M	M	M	M	M	M
Osteoporosis	M	M	M	M	M	M	M
Obesity	M	M	m	M	M	M	M
PMS	M	M	M	M	M	M	M
Phlebitis	M	M	M	M	M	M	M
Parasites	M	M	M	M	M	C	M
Parkinson's Disease	M	M	M	M	M	M	M
Strokes	M	M	M	M	M	M	M
Ulcers	M	M	M	M	M	M	M
Yeast Infection	M	M	M	M	M	C	M

**Virtually all chronic diseases involve some type of toxic condition. As discussed in the chapter on The Rite Toxin-free Living, toxins hamper the body's ability to function as designed.*

CHAPTER 1

BAD HABITS

Understanding Illnesses The Rite Way

Betty, a large, elegantly dressed woman with sparkling brown eyes and cafe-au-lait skin, sighed as she sank into a chair across from my desk. "With more than 500 employees to manage," she said, "I've already got the weight of the world on my shoulders. And I'll be damned," she added, pointing to her hips and giving me a wry smile, "if I'm going to carry it *here*."

Betty was, in fact, carrying over 200 pounds on her 5'8" frame. And at only 46 years old, she had become diabetic. "I like spending money on clothes," she said, "but not because I can't fit into what I just bought four months ago. I've got to lose weight."

"And you've got to get healthy," I said. "Are you ready for that?" She assured me she was. That's when I interviewed her extensively about her lifestyle and eating habits. It was no wonder her body composition test revealed 45% percent body fat: She had been eating five donuts a day every day for the past twenty years!

"How do you feel about being a slave to this food?" I said.

"What do you mean? I'm not a slave to anything or anybody!"

I suggested she ponder that, and when she returned to my office the following week, she said that the thought of being a slave to any food had sparked a dedicated commitment within her to overcoming this habit. She followed my weight management program for about 8 months, losing nearly two pounds of fat per week until she reached her goal of 141 pounds,

22% body fat, and the elimination of all diabetic medications. She was no longer diabetic—and needed no drugs. Betty was clearly living The Rite Way.

You picked up this book, so you have most likely already sensed that there is something in the 7 Rite Rules that can help change your life. But before you can really change your life, you need to understand negative habits. Maybe, because of indulging poor habits and following a negative lifestyle for years, you feel trapped and in a rut. Some of you might even feel you've become a slave to various treatments, products, or drugs.

A number of theories explain why certain people are more prone than others to following negative lifestyles, whether it be overeating or drug abuse. Possible causes are said to include genetics, past lives, poor childhood training, imitating heroes, and others. Some of the more controversial theories include the idea that alcoholism, drug addictions, obesity, and compulsive sexual behaviors are for the most part derived from past life experiences.

This chapter deals forthrightly with the issue of denial and some of the proven methods used to help people raise their level of consciousness and begin to contemplate the possibilities of changing. While everyone can see the importance of breaking negative habits, this chapter also gives attention to the importance of initial and continued abstinence, including the practical realities of completely discontinuing a negative behavior.

"The greater the obstacle, the more glory in overcoming it."

—Moliere

If you believe you're ready to change your life and are ready to benefit from the 7 Rite Rules, read on. Even if you're afraid you might not be able to achieve your goals because of deeply ingrained negative habits, read on. And lastly, if you have friends or family or someone who is in need of life changes, The Rite Way is perfect if they're stuck and need help.

If you hold the view that you have a Soul and it is everlasting, then you may want to also consider the prospects of physical immortality. The key is for you to be of sound mind and body over the next few decades, as the probabilities for an everlasting body will increase substantially. The 7 Rite Rules will likely lead those who apply them to a salubrious centenarian status and beyond. However, the application of these rules is easier said than done. The vast majority of today's American population is, literally, a slave to some type of addiction, including lustful overeating, promiscuous indulgence in sexual activities, or indulgence in addictive substances such as tobacco, alcohol, sugar, cocaine, caffeine, sodas, processed foods, and prescription and recreational drugs. This same population relies on traditional medicine, heavy medication, unnecessary surgeries, and a systemic lifestyle of stress, rushing, and negative feelings with no thought to energy, purity, hydration, or any number of healthful, life-improving nutrients. Following the 7 Rite Rules will grant you the health and vitality you will need to live longer, and to be there when new energy and medical developments are ready to be applied for limitless life extensions.

Overcoming Bad Habits Is a Major Challenge

During three years of research, writing, and publishing a Ph.D. dissertation on Personal Health Management, I came to the troubling conclusion that summarily telling patients what to do to overcome chronic illnesses is not enough. There is a syndrome generally called "engrained bad habits" that is behind negative behaviors and lifestyles. These negative lifestyles, in turn, are primarily responsible for the great number of today's chronic health disorders. Over the past 15 years in clinical practice and in an abundance of research by many institutions, others have come to see what I've long known: Most patients, if only told what to do to correct a chronic lifestyle disorder, will most likely not comply on a long-term basis. They may have the best of intentions while visiting with the doctor, but once out into the real world, where they face all of the same surroundings and people on a daily basis, most will have severe difficulty complying.

Innumerable Bad Habits, Innumerable Supposed Causes

Yogananda Paramahansa, considered a Master of wisdom by those who have known him, said in one of his many lectures, "the greatest obstacle to happiness is our bad habits. Habit can be both beneficial and our worst enemy. Bad habits will make not only you but everyone around you uncomfortable whereas your good habits will be a joy to you and to others also."

Yogananda's remarks, although simply stated, are packed with much wisdom and supported by considerable research and direct clinical experience in helping patients overcome negative habits. Here are some of my findings: Habits are formed gradually, by repetition of an action. Some claim that it may take about seven years to firmly establish a bad habit. I believe it often occurs more rapidly, especially in childhood when the mind is more pliable.

Numerous theories attempt to describe and explain what drives people to behave in ways that are obviously destructive to their health and well-being. The Bible even weighs in, making the case in the Adam and Eve story that one should not indulge in a negative behavior in the first place. Once the first indulgence is performed, this can be compared to an act of original sin, and now one is in the clutches of the devil and doomed to a life of repetitive negative behaviors.

The Body Is Like a Robot, Following Mind Grooves

The concept of a pliable subconscious mind posits that grooves are formed with increasing depth with each repetition of a particular behavior. The idea of "mind grooves" is a metaphor used quite often in the literature to describe habit formation. The pliability of the subconscious mind, during the formative years, tends to make for deeper grooves with repetitive behavior. This is not a problem when the groove results in a good habit and does not require changing. On the other hand, when a bad habit is formed, particularly during childhood, there is more time to increase the depth of the groove and this presents more of a challenge when change is desired during adulthood. The theory, from a behavioral standpoint, is that the body is comparable to a robot and will do whatever the mind tells it to do. When grooves are deep enough in the subconscious mind, the body develops tendencies that are expressed in the form of good and bad habits.

Of course good and bad habits can also be developed during adulthood but, as a rule, more time is required to develop grooves with depth because the subconscious mind becomes less pliable and more rigid with age.

Bad Habits Can Be Compared to an Octopus

Comparing the effects of bad habits to an octopus with many tentacles that can easily hold you in its grasp is another useful metaphor for bad habits. Once the tentacles hold sway, they can induce humans to behave like slaves by holding them in the clutches of many-armed forces and thereby continuously maintain the desire to engage in repetitive negative behaviors. Instead of a groove getting deeper, as in the previous analogy, every time you engage in a negative behavior another tentacle adds its force to keep you in the grasp of the habit.

The Heredity Theory

Other beliefs point to heredity as the most likely cause of many addictive behaviors, such as obesity, alcoholism, and drug abuse. In other words, some research implies that a fat gene may be responsible for obesity and that overeating is beyond the control of those obese individuals. Or maybe an alcohol-dependence gene is inherited from the mother or father that gives offspring a propensity for alcohol dependence. The list is nearly endless for the responsibilities laid upon the mother and/or father as the cause for the ill behaviors of their children.

The genes inherited from our parents are certainly important in building and maintaining our sacred bodies, but surprisingly many prominent researchers have verified that genetics are responsible for less than one-half percent of all chronic diseases. While many diseases such as sickle cell anemia and Huntington's disease are truly genetic diseases, many people have been overly influenced by the heavy media coverage and have attributed genes as a cause of many chronic illnesses that aren't truly genetically based. Even with a genetic component, lifestyle is a much more important factor when it comes to chronic diseases.

The Theories of Karma and Past Lives as the Cause of Bad Habits

There is also a theory that goes beyond the parents supplying an ill gene, and implicates past lives or incarnations of the Soul as having a karmic and dominant effect on the present incarnation and behaviors.

While the Western mindset, by and large, does not accept the proposition of reincarnation, the vast majority of the Eastern world embraces reincarnation as a natural cycle for all beings. What most people do not know is that up until 500 AD nearly the whole civilized world held the view that reincarnation was in fact part of the natural cycle of the Soul. However, documented history tells us that the Eastern Pope Justinian, located in Constantinople, Turkey, held a special meeting of Bishops and Cardinals and decreed that Christianity would now teach that the Soul does not exist until conception. He further decreed that the Soul only exists in the present body and when the body dies, the Soul either goes to Hell or Heaven and remains there forever.

Justinian believed that this new position gave the church much more leverage and control over its population. He felt that having the practitioners believe the present life was the only life would make them more likely to conform to the wishes of the church and refrain from doing bad things. Justinian also banished the concept of *karma,* which means "what you sow in this life you shall also reap in the next incarnation of your Soul."

Ironically the concept of karma and reincarnation, if properly understood by the masses, should have a most profound effect on behavior in the here and now. But Justinian did not see it as an effective deterrent to negative behaviors in the present, because he viewed reincarnation as opportunity for redeeming one's Soul in the future. Therefore, if some finality could be brought to bear on the present life with banishment to Hell, offering no chance for redemption after death, the church would surely have more control of the practitioners' sinful behavior.

While the concept of reincarnation does offer opportunities for redemption in the subsequent life of the Soul, it also carries with it the karma from the previous life that will now have to be dealt with in the new life. For example, the karmic idea is that alcoholism, obesity, sexual addiction, and other diseases, as well as cravings and propensities are related to actions or deeds in a previous life. Some scientists and philosophers describe these diseased conditions as part of the DNA inherent in the genes of the parents and passed on to the children. But many esoterists and Masters of ageless wisdom claim that Souls carry permanent atoms that record all habits, propensities, and cravings, and these are carried from incarnation to incarnation until the Soul learns to overcome them.

Negative Energy and Consciousness Can Cause Bad Habits

Dr. David Hawkins offers another concept for describing bad habit propensities in his book *Power vs. Force*. He defines a well-recognized set of attitudes and emotions that are linked to specific attractor energy fields, similar to electromagnetic fields gathering iron filings. For example, levels of consciousness with energy ratings of shame, guilt, apathy, grief, fear, desire, and anger all attract the establishment of negative habits.

His ratings are based on kinesiology testing, which is the study of muscles and their movements. Holistic doctors and chiropractors have been conducting this type of testing and research for more than 20 years to determine the physical condition of patients and likely causes of chronic illnesses.

In general, a typical test could be performed as follows:

1. The subject stands erect with right arm relaxed at his side, left arm extended parallel to the floor.
2. The tester faces the subject and places left hand on subject's right shoulder and tester places right hand on subject's extended left arm just above the wrist.
3. The subject is told to resist while the tester pushes down on the extended left arm and asks the subject to say what his name is. The subject's arm will stay straight and not move down providing the right name is given.
4. The tester asks the subject to say his name is something other than what it is while pushing down on his left arm and the tester finds the subject's left arm going weak and down with an untrue statement.

Although this is a simplified description of the kinesiology testing process, it supplies the basics for how truth and falsity can be determined in response to specific declarative statements. Many health practitioners use this testing technique to determine what may be the cause of specific symptoms or illnesses.

Dr. Hawkins, however, as an M.D. and psychiatrist has taken this science to new levels by proving that kinesiology testing can also be used to determine emotional levels with a great deal of accuracy. Simply put, those with a consciousness level below 200 are prone to developing destructive habits.

After many years of testing thousands of people with kinesiology methods, Dr. Hawkins was able to attach a power rating to each level of consciousness. For example, shame is given a rating at a level of 20, guilt at 30, apathy at 50, grief at 75, fear at 100, desire at 125, anger at 150, and pride at 175. Dr. Hawkins contends that nearly 80 percent of the population has a consciousness level below 200, and this could offer an explanation as to why vast numbers of people are struggling with the chains of bad habits.

The encouraging aspect of all this research into propensities for behavior is that they are all correctable. Some of the theories presented here include both physical and spiritual, suggesting a raising of consciousness to levels of enlightenment where one realizes he or she is actually the Soul and the body may be only a temporary vehicle. When one sees the light of this concept all things are possible, including the curing of all physical diseases like obesity, alcoholism, sexual addictions, and other lifestyle problems.

Controversial, but Non-Offensive Causes of Disease

Many are offended when I refer to chronic diseases and include homosexuality. Certainly there is controversy in labeling it as a disease. It's certainly one of several sexual issues that, examined in an objective way, is in the full and literal sense for many who face it a "dis-ease." As with some heterosexuals, many homosexuals feel they are consumed and in many respects driven by an obsessive sexual urge.

It's similar to many of the terms obese patients use when they describe being driven by compulsive overeating urges, and by alcoholics who cannot resist the urge to drink. In heterosexuals, many are driven to compulsive promiscuous sexual activities.

However, there are additional factors I'd like shine light on regarding the differences between homosexual males and others (women and men) suffering from the problems of compulsive sex. The heterosexual male is driven to engage in natural acts of sex as designed by divine intelligence. While it may be excessive, the practice is part of the programmed male urge to propagate. From a holistic standpoint, one where the body is held sacred and pure, a male homosexual engaging in the sex act is considered to be violating nature's design for the body's delicate chemical balance and immune system.

Why do I describe the male homosexual position as a potentially negative one? While it's true that compulsive sexual behavior exists in heterosexual males (and homo- and heterosexual females, as well), male homosexuals have a more difficult karmic birthright to contend with. As with many habits in our lives (negative and positive alike), we are born with them. Past lives, past cultures, and past lifestyles have accumulated since ancient times and for many, the sexual act has become compulsive. Physiologically, the body works in the way intended when a heterosexual male engages in sex with a woman. However, from a physical, chemical, and holistic energy perspective, the body is disrupted by the homosexual sexual act.

Males become the center of attention here because semen deposited in the colon repeatedly can cause a serious disruption of the immune system. The saline molecule within semen literally begins to destroy the major components of the immune system such as B and T cells, macrophages, and phagocytes. The saline solution works fine in the vaginal canal of a female in that it protects the sperm from being killed by her immune system. However, the same solution in the intestinal system, where 60 percent of the immune system resides, causes interference and seriously weakens overall defenses.

Some may wonder what caused a heterosexual in a past life to engage in homosexual behavior in the first place. An interesting account of this is given by the Tibetan Master Djwhal Khul, in the book *Esoteric Healing*. He describes a condition that has its roots in the Lemurian civilization, which existed several hundred thousand years ago. Homosexuality is what is called a "left-over" from sexual excesses of Lemurian times. Khul's contention is that homosexuality is not inherited genetically from your mother or father but from the physical atom permanently attached to your Soul throughout all incarnations. Souls who individualized and incarnated in that vast period of time are the ones who today demonstrate homosexual tendencies. In those days, the sexual appetite was so urgent that the normal processes of human intercourse did not satisfy the insatiable desires of the advanced man of that period. According to Khul, Soul force, flowing in through the processes of individualization, served to stimulate the lowest centers. Hence forbidden methods were practiced. Thus those who practiced them are today, in great numbers, in incarnation, and the ancient habits are too strong for them. However, Khul says individuals today should be far enough advanced upon the evolutionary path so that the ability to change lies ready for them at this time—if they choose to employ it.

While the preceding explanation for homosexuality covers the cause for the vast majority of homosexuals, Khul points out that today there is also a form of imitative, or learned, homosexuality. A number of persons of all classes may tend to imitate their perceived heroes—or people in society who they believe emulate behavior that is desirable or "cool." In other words, they were not born with a predisposition to the act. Moreover, Khul claims that imitative behavior is one of the prevalent reasons why many men and women today engage in homosexual activities, and is based upon a too-active imagination, plus a powerful physical or sexual nature, and prurient curiosity. This category accounts for much, but not most, of the homosexual and lesbian "dis-ease" that some may feel.

Bad Habits Can Stem from Imitating Others

Today's sociologists and psychologists believe many people who take the first step into addictive behaviors, such as tobacco, caffeine, and other drugs, start with the desire to imitate the people they look up to. It may be as simple as believing that the person who engages in the activity is somehow better or has achieved a higher status in life. A prime example is the entire class of Americans who began smoking in the 30s and 40s because they saw movie stars looking glamorous on screen with lit cigarettes. What they didn't know was that they would acquire a debilitating habit, in most cases causing severe health problems, cancers, and death.

In either case, whether one brings a habit from a previous incarnation or acquires one in the present life, the effect of a negative lifestyle choice can be very debilitating and place the patient in a "dis-eased" condition for lengthy periods. It appears that the longer a habit is indulged, the more likely it is that it will dominate the personality and become an obsession or a compulsive disorder. Those who bring a habit from a previous life will have the largest challenges in overcoming it because the habit has had more time to develop. In the present life, those who develop habits during the formative years are likely to have more difficulty overcoming them than those developed during adulthood.

Why to Avoid the First Bad Step

One of the important lessons to be gained from this discussion should be to avoid taking the first step of any indulgence that could open the door to disease. An indulgence could be described as anything that could expose you to an addiction to which you might become enslaved. Many people scoff at the idea that forgoing a practice in the first place is too simplistic and unrealistic. However, when you give sufficient thought to dealing with the entire problem of bad habits, how they get started, and how to overcome them, prevention always gets the nod over cure. One of the best ways to instill the concept of prevention is through education of youth starting at a very young age.

Listening to the Wisdom of your Elders

This chapter covered a comprehensive list of negative habits. It talked about what they might be and how you might have acquired them. And while you may be feeling like this chapter only pointed out problems, the good news is that the 7 Rite Rules have to do with improving your life, purifying your body, and creating a healthy life. As I tell my patients, the hard work will pay off. The body can achieve immortality—physically—and the health of the body is a critical component influencing the everlasting state of the Soul. In the meantime, I leave you with a last note on stopping bad habits before they start: prevention.

Prevention is an area where the older members of our society—not just the elderly, but any older role model—can play an increased role in serving the community by offering to help parents and their children see the wisdom of prevention. Conventional wisdom is that we learn about our mistakes by making them. A key aspect of prevention is that the elders in our society—parents, role models, doctors, professionals, and others—can guide the younger members away from taking that first step to forming bad habits.

Of course this continues to be the major theme of this work. To prevent a disease is a much more desirable effort than to have to contend with all of the immensely challenging and costly curative measures. The next chapter strives to anchor further the importance of prevention by delineating many curative methods that have proven effective, but almost always are very challenging, time-consuming, and costly.

CHAPTER 2

THE RITE WAY TO CHANGE FOR LIFE

Wanting to Change Is the Key to Wellness and Longevity

Like many smokers, Colleen wanted to quit but couldn't find the strength to stick with it. In the dozen or so times she had tried to kick the habit, she had never been able to abstain for more than a week. Then, she learned that several of her friends had successfully quit with my help, and she arrived at my clinic ready to get started with hypnotherapy.

"I'll never do it on my own," she said, "I'm a TV actress, and with seventy-five percent of the crew lighting up, not to mention the stress and long hours, I don't have a chance. But I don't want to go like my father did. Lung cancer. Smoked a pack a day, just like me. I've been doing that for 18 years; he did it for 35." Colleen sighed and flipped back her long, blonde hair. "Besides," she said, pointing to her face, "My living depends on this. Between you and me, I'm 37, but I'm supposed to be a lot younger. And cigarettes aren't exactly helping my skin maintain the illusion."

When I told Colleen that pre-testing indicated she was not yet ready to rush into hypnotherapy, she was disappointed. But I insisted we first had to work on properly developing a conscientious commitment through contemplation and planning. Otherwise, she would greatly reduce her chances of success. It was hard for her to put off the hypnotherapy, but Colleen agreed to do the necessary preparatory work first. It paid off. At the time of this writing, she has been nicotine free for five years. And at age 42, she looks younger and feels better than she did at 37. Colleen is living The Rite Way.

Whereas Chapter 1 dealt with how bad habits are formed, here the focus is on how to overcome bad habits and effect permanent change. Like Colleen, you need to be prepared so the 7 Rite Rules can be followed effectively. The modern methods for change require recognizing and implementing a six-stage process in order to effect successful habit changes. I've taught my patients the six steps for many years and it's the same one that several Ph.D.s have formalized in a book on the process.

In broad terms, the process includes the following six stages:

1. Pre-contemplation
2. Contemplation
3. Planning
4. Action
5. Maintenance
6. Termination

It's important that you follow each step in proper sequence. For example, research has shown that those who go directly from contemplation to action, bypassing the planning stage, almost always are unsuccessful and the entire process has to be repeated. Examining each step with more detail we find that pre-contemplation is actually a form of denial that requires the subject to become aware, or raise their consciousness, to understand the problem exists. This requires understanding the self-defeating defenses that get in the way of recognizing that a problem even exists.

Contemplation primarily involves seeking out more information, more awareness, and more self-motivation. The planning stage is the cornerstone for effective action and affords the opportunity to make a solid commitment to behavior change. It includes delineating specific steps that will be taken to solve the problem during the action stage.

The action stage requires an active commitment to change. The focus is on the process of control, including use of several techniques such as rewards, replacement, and helping relationships. The maintenance stage is often the most challenging in that successful change means change sustained over long periods of time, perhaps several years. Two factors are fundamental to successful maintenance: sustained, long-term effort and a revised lifestyle. The last state, termination, is reached when one no longer has to think about the negative habit that existed previously.

Within each stage there are particular processes and techniques essential to effect movement from one stage to the next.

For example, many people who have problems with food are quite literally slaves to their sense of taste, and the thought of being free is not part of their thinking process. They can generally be described as being in a state of denial with an inability to recognize any type of problem or consequence created by their behavior, even though they might be aware of obesity-related diseases such as diabetes. Based on whatever toxic, pre-packaged food product that appeals to their taste that moment, or hour, or day, they could be committing suicide, only on a different time table, every bit as much as someone ingesting arsenic.

Prevention of Poor Habits and Chronic Illnesses

As humans, we take our miraculous physical bodies for granted. We forget the importance of taking proper care of these amazing organic machines. However, the inherent wisdom of our very bodies, or body intelligence, is that if cared for properly, we can prevent or eliminate virtually all chronic diseases. We can achieve this state of healthfulness if we raise our consciousness and understand the need to put our bodies first. This healthfulness is what can ultimately lead to a longevity that medical science can prolong, what I call making the prospect of "immortality" a reality.

Most people go to a doctor to be treated for their ills without thinking about the need for themselves to somehow change their lifestyles or mindsets. They think about curing the disease or condition but give no thought to what caused it. Although it should be common sense to follow the advice of their physician, few people take responsibility for their own lives even after being told by an expert that change is necessary.

How does one get to the place where they realize over-consumption and do-nothing sedentarianism are habitual conditions that must be corrected if health and longevity are to be achieved? The raising of consciousness to prevent diseases, and the challenging process of overcoming poor habits, are in fact the major health issues facing the vast majority of the population.

Who's in Charge...the Mind, Body, or Soul?

When asking "what is the essence of life?" the concept of "the Soul" often enters the picture. Wise men, such as sages and Masters, have written that when the Soul is in the body of one who is immersed in low levels of consciousness and dominated by poor habits, it is much like a captain who has lost control of his ship to drunken sailors. To the extent that the personality drives the human body to violate and override its natural beauty and wisdom, the Soul unfortunately may just go along for the ride until the next incarnation. Referring again to Yogananda's writings, he says "you do not know what good or bad habits you have established in previous lives and you should be conscious about what you do in this life, lest the slightest stimulus gives a fresh hold to some bad habits that have been trailing you through incarnations." This could explain how it happens that a person may take just one drink, and his old habit of former lives awakens, and he is snared into the grips of alcoholism in this present life.

"The only thing worse than having no sight is having no vision."

—Helen Keller

In reviewing the vision and insights of a fair number of ancient Masters, one of the key points to remember is that we as human beings do not just consist of our bodies. In reality, we are Souls occupying miraculous physical coverings called bodies that allow us to function on Earth. These wonderful physical bodies in fact do not require much attention and will function perfectly so long as we follow some physical and metaphysical guidelines, what I call the 7 Rite Rules.

If you follow the 7 Rite Rules, you will develop a bodily rhythm that will lead to resonation of the Soul, enhancing the health and vitality of the body. The establishment of this rhythm is essential for the prevention of illnesses and for the effective changing of lifestyles that can only be accomplished when one gains control of the body. Once you can overcome bad habits, you have a strong indication that you can, in fact, gain control over your entire body.

Don't Give a Bad Habit a Chance to Get Started

As trite and obvious as that advice may seem to be, it is worthwhile re-emphasizing that prevention is the most effective method for dealing with the problem of poor habits. I realize much of what I'm telling you sounds very obvious and repetitive, but it's only because I understand that correcting poor habits is one of the most challenging of all health endeavors. So challenging, in fact, that I think it's worth paying attention to the wisdom of the ages that underlines the importance of prevention.

> *"Where there's a will, there's a way."*
>
> —Anonymous

The most prudent rule to follow in prevention is to avoid exposing the body to the majority of processed products, whether man-made or natural. This includes not only pre-packaged, highly processed items, but also items produced or distilled from natural sources such as alcohol, tobacco, or other drugs. Alcohol may be distilled from natural fruits and grains, but it's still processed. Tobacco is cured, cocaine is synthesized, and even coffee beans are leached and roasted. Fresh fruits and vegetables, seeds, nuts, and sprouted grains require no processing. Another example of being ensnared with first-time exposure includes the consumption of products containing additives such as sugar. Consumption of these feel-good-taste-good products can easily be the start of a craving for sweets, leading to a lifetime of serious negative health consequences as adults. There will be will plenty of examples furnished later to spell out addictions associated with processed foods that were once natural.

Another way to view the concept of prevention and how powerful and influential it can be is to realize that in addition to benefiting your own life, you will be setting an excellent example for those around you. In terms of service to the community and humanity there is no better way serve than by setting proper lifestyle examples.

Don't Mix with Those Who Have Bad Habits

Yogananda offers additional good advice when he says, "if you have a particular poor habit it would be prudent to not mix with those who have the same kind of bad habit. If you have a desire to smoke or drink for example, it would be best to avoid those who have those habits." There is some truth to the adage that "people who support your bad habits are not really your friends." For example, if you are trying to quit smoking, it may be hard for you to spend time with your friends who insist on lighting up. If you are trying to give up caffeine, it might be difficult for a while to meet with your book group at your local coffee shop.

As parents, we try to educate our children about avoiding bad habits in their school years. Influenced by other children, they feel little choice if they don't join the crowd smoking or drinking. They fear they might be ostracized. Peer pressure can be immense and significantly influence choices children make. Acknowledging this condition, parents should spend extra effort on talking, training, and setting proper examples. Even children should be introduced to spiritual concepts and taught to resist bad habits, especially when it comes to food and drink temptations.

Repetition: A Tool for Preventing Bad Habits

Adults should not only set proper examples for children, but also indoctrinate them on the nature of bad habits through repetitive instructions. It is appropriate to use metaphors described in the previous chapter that depict bad habits as monsters or animals like an octopus with many tentacles to hold you in their grasp. Once they entrap you, those octopus tentacles can feed on you and virtually drain you of your will to fight and live a healthy lifestyle. The more personal and vivid the analogy, the more likely it is to have a lasting impact on the consciousness of the child.

Many Masters through the ages have made the point that a slave is a slave. No matter who you have to answer to, whether another human, food, drink, or drug… you're a slave! If it is something you are craving to satisfy your senses, you are a slave to it. What pleases your taste does not always satisfy the needs of your body. If you could actually see the body's complex wisdom in dynamic action, you would not want to take part in any negative action that could impede this divine power.

Masters like Yogananda have emphasized that many Americans are heavy meat-eaters and neglect fresh fruits and vegetables in their diet. In many respects, they are addicted to meat and as a result, their kidneys and intestines are at high risk for blockages and cancerous growths. However, most of my patients have the same reaction when I suggest they give up meat to help reduce cardiovascular risks or some forms of cancer: "I'd rather be dead than to have to give up meat." When one reflects on the real meaning of this kind of statement, it begs the question: Are you a slave to your bad habits? If giving up meat was truly best for your body, wouldn't you really want to do it? Admitting that you can't get along without consuming a certain food, drink, or even medication automatically puts you in the category of "slave."

Dare to Take the Slave Test?

Are you a slave? As an interesting test, make a list of your favorite foods, even just the foods you really like. Try giving up each of those favorites for two to three weeks. You'll find many redeeming benefits to this type of "at will" abstinence. One is the feeling of power you will recognize when you develop that physical and mental "won't power" you can maintain no matter how you are urged or tempted. The level of consciousness required to accomplish this "won't power" is labeled as "courage" and has a rating of 200 on Dr. Hawkins' scale, as described in the previous chapter.

Ancient Ways to Create and Destroy Habits

Many Masters and yogis advocate that when you want to create a good habit or destroy a bad habit, you should concentrate on the brain cells, the storehouse of the mechanism of habits. One of the ancient ways teachers advocate for creating a good habit is to meditate on the center between the eyebrows, deeply affirming the good habit you want to install. This affirmation process can be highly effective, especially when it takes the form of a mantra that is repeated many times over as described later in the chapter.

Mediation can help you overcome bad habits. When meditating, you should focus your concentration and visualize, erasing or paving over the bad habit grooves. The example of grooves with references to bad habits is a popular metaphor used among Masters who speak to the problem of overcoming bad habits. Many of them have the power of clairvoyance and can literally see physical groove manifestations where others cannot. Many of my patients speak about their cravings with words such as "I feel like I am in a rut" and "the same recording keeps repeating itself over and over." Visualize a groove in the mind and concentrate on virtually covering the groove of whatever bad habit is being attacked, and your chances of success can be greatly enhanced.

At this point I am going to go beyond the wisdom of the ages and discuss some of the more recent developments and methodologies proven to be effective for removing poor habits and changing from undesirable lifestyles to positive lifestyles.

Recognizing the Stages in the Change Process

Many people with bad habits, addictions, or health problems may or may not want to change. They often have found ways to rationalize, ignore, or view their condition as a non-problem. Psychologists generally label behavior of this type "denial," meaning a mental state where one refuses to acknowledge that a problem exists. In their book, *Changing for Good*, doctors Prochaska, Norcross, and DiClemente label the denial process as one of "pre-contemplation." According to them, pre-contemplation is the first of six well-defined steps in every change process. The five other steps of change following pre-contemplation are contemplation, preparation, action, maintenance, and termination. They developed this concept of six stages after interviewing a large sample of people who were involved in change and those who were considered successful changers. My experiences with thousands of patients fit almost perfectly with the descriptions assigned to the six-step stages of change. Additionally, I've found their description of change processes and techniques can be assigned to specific stages and are remarkably constant from one person to the next regardless of the problem.

Getting Past the Denial State Is the Biggest Challenge

The chances are fairly good that readers of this book are not in a serious state of denial. I can make this assumption because people in the stage of denial or pre-contemplation refuse to think about their condition. They typically go to extremes to avoid exposure to any information or communication that may speak to the negative aspects of their particular addiction. If, for example, a television program begins to talk about their kind of problem they will leave the room or change the channel. If a newspaper or magazine features stories about their habits they will refuse to read them. Why? Because if they haven't consciously admitted to their problem, then subconsciously they don't want to be reminded that a change may be necessary. This stage of denial can also be explained by employing the cognitive dissonance concept. Patients may only be cognitive of information that supports their plight and makes them feel justified and comfortable. For example, heavy alcohol drinkers will immediately latch on to a report that indicates a drink or two a day helps prevent heart attacks. All other negative information about alcohol does not resonate or is not recognized as applicable to them. If they are confronted with the problem, typically their response will be one of rationalization, denying they have a problem, or citing their faulty research.

Courage Is Required to Get Past Denial

Generally, all of us find that denial is what holds us in the pre-contemplation stage. People in this stage usually deny responsibility in order to avoid punishment when they are accused of doing something wrong, particularly if they enjoy their negative behavior or bad habit, such as someone who smokes cigarettes. Sometimes they might admit to the bad habit but rationalize their actions. They'll use any justification to defeat themselves and in many respects they fight hard to stay in the denial stage. The struggle continues because it feels safe. They can't fail in this state. In a sense, pre-contemplators are free from social pressures when they create awkward scenes in order to convince those who care about them that they really don't want to discuss the situation. Some of those in denial are so negative that they have become resigned to their fate, using a hopeless mindset. They often believe that merely thinking of change is to risk failure again. Defeatism dominates their thoughts and they have given up on any prospect of changing. With this attitude, many in this early stage can be described as having given up on themselves. They are so habituated to the fog and density of their plight that they are oblivious to its existence, regarding it as right and good with the unchangeable place of their daily life.

Getting Out of the Stage of Denial

Some claim that elevating one to the stage of contemplation may be an inscrutable or mysterious process. No one really knows what causes a person to feel the need to make a change. Perhaps it could have a spiritual connection to a prayer or meditation, in essence helping them "see the light" or the error of their ways. Some tell of experiences with self-help groups or hearing an inspirational anecdotal story from a member. Others point to some definable incident that moved them to reflect on their condition as a possible problem. Maybe they or a family member experienced an event such as a birth or death in the family, or possibly an emergency visit to a hospital, or a geographical change, a loss of job, or gaining a new relationship. Any of these events could spark an awakening of the consciousness and an awareness that a change of habits might bring some happiness and/or improvement to their life.

"History has demonstrated that the most notable winners usually encountered heartbreaking obstacles before they triumphed. They won because they refused to become discouraged by their defeats."

—B.C. Forbes

On the other hand, you should be aware that often there is another pattern. If the negative lifestyle choice is an addiction, often the addict has to fail dismally, or hit bottom, before seeing the light. Helpers can be a key factor in assisting an addict to see the light, but many times in the process of trying to help a loved one the helper is taken advantage of. In some cases helpers are emotionally, physically, and monetarily dragged down and left utterly and continuously frustrated in unsuccessful attempts to force a person to see reason.

Helpers who develop a "tough love" attitude toward the pre-contemplator work best. Helpers should be encouraged to address specific disruptive and distressing behavior with some of the following techniques:

1. Ensure that each negative behavior is followed by a consistent consequence.
2. Insist that the pre-contemplator accept responsibility for actions.
3. Frequently and directly recommend behavior change by encouraging an appointment with a professional.

Many programs are available to help people overcome bad habits, but they are all directed at those who are ready to make a change. According to several studies, fewer than 20 percent of any problem population is prepared to move to the next stage. What that means to you is that fewer than 20 of 100 people with, say, a weight problem, are driven to make a change in their life and address it. However, once the problem has been acknowledged, a person moves to the next stage of change: contemplation. No matter how ready you might be to break your habit and move directly to the action stage, we know from research it will lower your chance for success. Therefore, it is inappropriate to encourage one to move directly into the action stage and bypass the contemplation or planning stage.

Contemplation: Measuring the Pros and Cons of your Change

Several principles, processes, and techniques are recommended to help people through these stages. For example, the first principle of progress in helping people advance from pre-contemplation to contemplation is to increase the perception of the benefits of changing the problem behavior. Based on my experience with patients perceived to be in a state of denial, when they visit me for a consultation, I will present as much beneficial (pro) information as possible in dramatic fashion while I have their attention.

In Dr. Prochaska's book *Changing for Good,* he finds that in moving from the stage of pre-contemplation to contemplation, the perceived benefits of changing (pros) increase significantly and can be quantified. (See the following questionnaire.) Additionally, if one is to advance from contemplation to action, the perception of the negatives (cons) must decrease and this can also be quantified.

For example, when speaking to patient, here are some pros I give them, or reasons they should change: "If you will start thinking about and start planning for a weight management program, these are some of the benefits you can expect to receive":

1. You will be healthier.
2. Friends and relatives will feel better about you.
3. You will feel better about yourself.
4. You will function better.
5. You will be happier.
6. Your children will be better off because of the example you set.
7. You will worry less.
8. Friends and relatives will be happier when you change.

Then, I might ask them to think of reasons not to change. The idea behind this exercise is to decrease these "cons" at the contemplation stage of change so they don't come back to threaten success later. Here are some of the perceived cons to change from patients:

1. If I change, some people would think less of me.
2. It takes a lot of time.
3. I might fail.
4. It takes a lot of effort and energy.
5. I would have to give up some things I enjoy.
6. I would lose some benefits of my current behavior.
7. Other people would lose some benefits of my current behavior.
8. Some people would be uncomfortable.

Fill out the following questionnaire to see where you stand on the pros and cons of changing, and then add up your scores to see where you rate on Dr. Prochaska's scale.

Once you list these reasons (or others specific to your situation), you will rate them based on the level of importance.

QUESTIONNAIRE: PROS & CONS OF CHANGING

1=not important, 2=slightly important, 3=somewhat important
4=quite important, 5=extremely important

1. Some people would think less of me if I change		______
2. I would be healthier if I change	______	
3. Changing takes a lot of time		______
4. Some people would feel better about me if I change	______	
5. I'm concerned I might fail if I try to change		______
6. Changing would make me feel better about myself	______	
7. Changing takes a lot of effort and energy		______
8. I would function better if I change	______	
9. I would have to give up some things I enjoy		______
10. I would be happier if I change	______	
11. I get some benefits from my current behavior		______
12. Some people could be better off if I change	______	
13. Some people benefit from my current behavior		______
14. I would worry less if I change	______	
15. Some people would be uncomfortable if I change		______
16. Some people would be happier if I change	______	
	______	______
	PROS	CONS

Add up the scores on the odd-numbered items; this is the current score on the cons of changing. Add up the scores on the even items; this is the current score on the pros.

After adding up the score for both, look at your number.

Dr. Prochaska's findings indicate that 21 is an average pro and con score; therefore a pro score of 28 (one standard deviation) and a con score of less than 17 (.5 standard deviation) is necessary in order to show the contemplator is ready for the action stage.

Typically a mean score of 21 is found for the pros of changing pre-contemplators. Statistically it has been shown that a change of 7 points (one standard deviation) to a score of 28 is necessary in order to move to the next stage defined as contemplation.

Regarding the cons, for people in the contemplation stage, a score of 21 is typical and a decrease of 4 points (.5 standard deviation) has been found to be significant in order to be adequately prepared to move to the action stage. This quantification exercise may seem a bit confusing, but I believe that if you can persuade pre-contemplators to complete the real reasons they want to change, a meaningful dialogue will ensue.

In my lectures, I have found that a comparison to Plank's Quantum Theory on the behavior of sub-atomic particles can be useful in explaining what may be happening with humans regarding their changed behavior. With the quantum theory, Plank is basically postulating that only a quantum of energy—the smallest sub-atomic particle known—is needed to get other sub-atomic particles to change behavior and resonate or vibrate at higher levels. A quantum amount of energy, in sub-atomic parlance, virtually means very small, almost imperceptible differences of added energy are applied to a physical entity, but the effects can be pronounced. Quantums of energy can do very large tasks such as boil water and change metal color when heated. In a similar way, only a very small (quantum) amount of mental energy may be needed to spark human change.

With Dr. Prochaska's theory of measuring change, a movement of one standard deviation (or one point on a six-point bell curve) on the pro side and only .5 on the con side is sufficient to support a change in behavior. Once the individual has established readiness for action, additional processes and techniques can be used to help the person move to the next stage and eventually through the entire six levels.

Making a Commitment to Change

The major challenge in the entire change process has to do with getting people who are in a state of denial to recognize that a problem exists and to help them see that a change is necessary. The second most challenging part of the change process is getting to the action stage and staying in it. Staying in the action stage requires a clear commitment to change formed over a period of days and possibly weeks of contemplation and preparation. Intertwined into a commitment to make a change and move into the action stage is the process of consciousness raising, which is responsible for the positive results.

The concept of developing a bodily rhythm also comes into play, meaning success will ride on not just one area of your body or life, but all. This means that in making a decision to change one part of your life—such as losing weight or quitting a prescription drug—you must follow all of the seven wellness and longevity rules. When you develop a healthy mindset and rhythm, you will promote overall vitality and overcome not just one disorder like obesity, smoking, or drinking, but improve your overall life as well.

Staying in the Action Stage of Change

Once the commitment to change is made, there are many processes and techniques you can try to bolster your chances of success. You may even end up trying more than one over a set time period during the action stage, which in many cases may last for months. The processes that have been deemed effective during this stage include reprogramming, substitution, reward, control, and helping relationships.

How Affirmations Can Reprogram the Mind

Chapter 1 discussed the concept of bad habits being set in the subconscious mind like grooves in a record. These grooves need paving over and new good habit grooves need to be formed. I have found that the most effective results can be accomplished using a technique involving listening to repetitive affirmation messages. By listening to affirmative messages—in an active listening state for about 10 minutes before bedtime and in a passive state during the day—you will significantly reinforce your subconscious mind.

To use this technique, all that is required is to recite and record positive affirmations. I recommend using 100 or so. (The appendix contains a listing of affirmations for weight management and nutrition.) These can be recorded on disc or tape with one-beat-per-second background music for optimum subconscious reprogramming effect. If you don't like classical music, choose soothing music with the one-beat-per-second meter. No matter what your goal, tailor the affirmations to your situation and add new ones specific to the benefits in your own life.

Using your Affirmations with Breathing and Visualization

Once you've made your affirmation recording, you'll want to make sure you pair using it with breathing and visualization techniques. The best time to breathe, relax, listen to your affirmations, and visualize is just before bedtime.

Once you are in position, sitting on a chair or up in bed, relax by following a 7,1,7,1 nose breathing routine. In this routine, 7 counts of inhaling should be followed by 1 count of holding, followed by 7 counts of exhaling, followed by 1 count of holding. Repeat the process three times. Then visualize yourself as a successful changer. For example, if your affirmations are about your weight, imagine yourself in your best outfit or in a swimming suit at your target weight. Once you have visualized a successful image, consciously listen to at least 50 of the affirmations, which is about ten minutes' worth.

Sometime during the day, listen to another 50 affirmations—just let them play while getting ready for work or while driving in the car. No deep breathing or visualization is necessary while you follow this inactive listening process. The subconscious mind is hearing these messages and over a 21-day period, coupled with the evening attentive listening routine, a significant percentage of people will demonstrate positive change action.

There Are No Magic Bullets!

While I am very much enthused with the results experienced with the aforementioned affirmation process, it is important to remember that it does require a fair amount of commitment on the part of the patient to make this work effectively. I spend a good deal of time coaching the patient on the importance of making a habit out of listening to the affirmations. I may use another process termed "rewards" in order to help motivate regular listening by suggesting that patients "contract" with themselves, perhaps depositing $5 in a box every time the tape is played. I often suggest the reward and contracting process when I determine they want something costly as a reward—like new clothes or an appliance. Over a 21-day period this accumulation of dollars can serve as a powerful motivator for helping to reinforce the habit of listening to the affirmations. The affirmation process is not a "magic bullet." It doesn't work for everyone, however nearly 80 percent of the people who actually follow the 21-day listening routine claim fantastic results. If, for some reason, you're having problems following a regular pattern of listening, you're generally going to get less-defined results.

Negative versus Positive Power Effects of Affirmations

Why is the affirmation process so highly effective? Metaphorically the affirmation process can be viewed as reprogramming the subconscious computer, or building a new habit groove in the mind. It would also be appropriate to call it a form of self-hypnosis or positive thinking. Some believe it can be compared to the value of repeating a mantra that is used to help the meditation process. Others claim that it presents an excellent way to counter rigid and negative thought patterns that are common among those with poor habits. I have found that in addition to all of the above, it serves as an excellent way for building a positive rhythm into one's lifestyle in a relatively short period of time.

It is reasonable to question how a bad habit can be changed so quickly by the affirmation process. For example, how is a person who has overindulged a habit, such as consuming five or six cans of soda a day for 20 years, going to change just by listening to affirmations for 21 days? I like to think of it as the difference between multiplication and addition. The positive acts exponentially like multiplication, while the negative is only as strong as simple addition. Russian behavioral scientists came to this conclusion in the late 1950s after many years of researching the effects of affirmation training when coupled with baroque music. My clinical experience supports the notion that generally one negative event is about equal to one positive event. However, when positive events are grouped together they tend to display a synergistic exponential effect. For example, a power of 2 assigned to each positive event in a grouping of 10, 2 x 2 x 2 and so on, would amount to a total power of 1024, whereas a grouping of 10 negative events with a power of 2 each, 2 + 2 + 2 and so on, would amount to a total of 20.

What is the effect on the soda pop addict over a 20-year period who drinks six sodas a day, with 10 gulps per soda and each gulp rated as one negative event with a power of 2? All of these can be added up in terms of gulps for a total negative power of 876,000 over a 20-year period.

Using the power of 2 for each positive affirmation and applying the exponential effect, we can see that in a very short time (about 25 affirmations) the negative power of 876,000 can be easily exceeded.

Over a 21-day period of regularly listening to 100 affirmations a day, with background baroque music, the positive power number dwarfs the negative number and one can start to get a sense for why this process can be so powerful.

Substitution Is Another Effective Process

While the affirmation process is a highly effective change mechanism, others like "substitution" have also proven to be effective for supporting change during the action stage.

Researchers have found that when troubled behaviors are removed without providing substitutes, the risk of returning to old habits remains probable. The key here is to find substitute techniques that have proven effective over time. The following are techniques I often advocate for my weight management patients:

Exercise: It would be hard to find a more beneficial substitute for problem habits than physical exercise. The exercises specified in Chapter 8, "The Rite Rule # 6: Exercise," should be considered appropriate for a wide range of substitute behaviors. A combination of aerobic and anaerobic exercises such as bike riding, swimming, walking, weight lifting, rowing, and so on should be followed in a regular schedule. Among the many benefits of exercise is the production and release of hormones from the muscles into the bloodstream.

These hormones are called beta endorphins and they act as wonderful precursors for producing optimum levels of neurotransmitters in the brain. When neurotransmitters are at optimum levels there is a feeling of satisfaction and well-being, and generally the urge to indulge in negative behaviors is reduced or eliminated. For this reason alone, exercise should become a part of everyone's program for substituting good actions for bad.

Relaxation: In many instances exercise may not be appropriate to counter a problem. If a patient finds herself in a stressful work situation, for example, or feels the need for a cigarette, it may be difficult to substitute the urge with a bike ride or jog. In some cases, exercise won't work due to injury. In these kinds of cases, the relaxation technique can be considered an appropriate substitute for a problem behavior.

"The highest reward for a person's toil is not what they get for it, but what they become by it."

—John Ruskin

There are many popular ways to evoke a state of deep relaxation. Meditation, prayer, yoga, and deep breathing can all be used independently to achieve a state where the need to indulge in the problem behavior is reduced significantly. In a work environment my patients have found that the 7,1,7,1 deep breathing exercises are practical and effective and are rather easy to perform. Most communities offer classes on meditation and yoga and I highly recommend patients explore these techniques to determine if they may be helpful.

Environment Control: Another Effective Process

Unlike substitution, which involves changing the response to a given situation, environment control requires changing the situation itself. Environmental change involves restructuring the exposure to problem environments, making it less likely to stimulate a negative behavior.

One of the techniques used in environmental control is called avoidance. Many people think that they must rely on will power alone to fight temptation. But, avoidance is a key technique in the control process to help eliminate temptation. As Dr. Prochaska points out, avoidance should not be viewed as a sign of weakness or poor self-control, rather it should be looked at as effective self-control that prevents a problem from re-occurring. For example, if alcohol is a problem it makes sense to avoid keeping liquor in the house, or as Yogananda suggests, avoiding places and people who drink would certainly be helpful. Smokers should practice avoidance by removing cigarettes and ashtrays from their homes, and overeaters should not be bringing home problem foods.

Warning Sign Awareness: As you become more aware of your environment, you'll find you're on the lookout for cues or warning signs that may trigger problem behaviors. As you become aware of these warning signs, you can also begin to make plans for how to deal with what they signal. Dr. Prochaska points out the idea here is to gradually expose yourself to the warning signs by role-playing in your imagination, imagining a positive response as you progress through the action stage. Practicing how you will respond to the warning signs will gradually increase your resistance when the real situation occurs. For example, if you are an overeater, and you know you will be attending an affair where a great deal food will be served, you should develop a plan in advance as to how you will appropriately respond to the situation. If you feel you are not ready for that kind of environment, then it may be best to avoid this sort of affair until you gain more confidence in the action stage.

Reminders to Help Stay on Course

You can use a number of simple techniques to remind yourself about the pitfalls and warning signs during the action stage. Something as simple as a NO SMOKING sign on your desk or a STOP sign on the refrigerator door can be very effective. Dr. Prochaska claims that although this type of reminder may seem artificial and unnatural, it should be viewed like stop signs at a busy intersection, and therefore useful for controlling behavior.

I encourage my patients to make use of one of the most effective reminders in the form of a weekly "To Do List." A list of action goals could include the following:

1. Monday, take a half hour walk at 7:30 a.m.
2. Tuesday, exercise with weights for 25 minutes at 5:30 p.m.
3. Wednesday, 15 minutes of quiet time or meditation at 12:45 p.m.
4. Thursday, take half hour walk at 7:30 a.m.
5. Friday, 15 minutes of quiet time or yoga at 12:45 p.m.
6. Saturday, 25 minutes of weight exercises at 8:00 a.m.
7. Sunday, take half hour walk at 8:00 a.m.

Of course this action list could be incorporated with other activities like shopping, errands, and so on, but one of the major benefits in the action stage is in the form of positive reinforcement gained from simply checking off each action item after it has been completed.

The Process of Rewards Can Be Highly Effective

In making a list, there is the reinforcement benefit that comes from simply checking off each action as completed. There can also be a powerful psychological reward that can come from vocally reaffirming what a good thing you just did by immediately congratulating yourself with "Nice job, I knew I could do it," or "Keep up the good work." These healthy feedback pat-on-the-back rewards are not to be underestimated. They are the corollary to reprogramming the subconscious mind by listening to repetitive positive affirmations on tape as described earlier.

Dr. Prochaska claims that historically, rewards have been used to reinforce desirable behaviors, and punishments used to discourage undesirable ones. However, most experienced behavioral psychologists now believe that punishment tends to suppress troubled behavior only temporarily, and therefore rewards should be the process of choice. I emphatically support this position and I tell all of my patients who are seeking change that the subconscious mind is always listening. If you make negative statements like "how could I be so stupid," or "I'm really dumb," or "I must be crazy," these are recorded in the subconscious mind and serve to undermine the accomplishment of positive change.

Rewards can also be effective in physical form during the action stage. Personalized agreements with oneself can be excellent motivators for helping to accomplish goals. Written contracts tend to be more powerful than spoken ones so, for example, you could write down that for every pound lost you will pay yourself $10, putting the money toward a substantial purchase after a certain amount of weight loss.

It is best when patients recognize that rewards can also be given for not engaging in problem behavior, and that it would also be appropriate to reward yourself for substituting a healthier alternative. In your contract with yourself, you could add another clause where you would pay yourself $5 for every 30 minutes spent exercising. As Dr. Prochaska states, "It is often easier to promote a new behavior than to eliminate an old one, and, as we have seen, substitution is a key process to self-change."

Helping Relationships During the Action Stage

Most successful changers have found ways to enlist the help of family or friends to bear the challenge of change during the action stage. During the preparation stage it would be appropriate to share your burden by going public and discussing your plans and goals with significant others in your life. It would be best to let people know that even if you become anxious, irritable, confused, or difficult, you want and need their support.

Ask Someone to Be your Buddy: There are times when two people, working as a team, are able to change themselves more effectively than either can alone. Running, walking, swimming, biking, and so on are easier and more fun with a loved one or a friend. It is appropriate to ask one or more of your helpers to join you in your substituting techniques. It is also appropriate to elicit rewards from helpers for even small amounts of progress. It's okay to tell your helpers that "strokes" come in many forms and that they can brag about your progress, give extra hugs, small presents, even back massages, all appreciated as useful rewards.

Keep Helping Relationships Positive: Sometimes family members are silent supporters for many days of progress, but become vocal critics when you slip up. It is best to tell them up front that reinforcement is superior to punishment in promoting behavior change, and that scolding, nagging, and preaching are not forms of support, even if they are well intentioned.

If you don't have anyone immediately available to call on as a support helper, it is highly recommended that those actively seeking change find a local support group. People facing the same problems can reinforce and help support you through the tough periods and remind you of the benefits of changing. In most communities you can find a wide array of support groups, such as Alcoholics Anonymous, Overeaters Anonymous, Smokers Anonymous, Gamblers Anonymous, and many others through newspaper, churches, or health care providers.

Dr. Hawkins reminds us in his book *Power vs. Force* that in every study of recovery from hopelessness there has been a major shift in consciousness, so that the attractor patterns that resulted in the bad habit no longer dominated. The steps necessary for recovery of millions of people suggests that the 12-step process has merit. Carl Jung's advice is "Throw yourself wholeheartedly into any spiritual group that appeals to you whether you believe in it or not and hope that in your case a miracle may occur." The power of helping relationships should not be underestimated; they are of vital importance during the action stage and every effort should be made to seek out and establish these relationships.

The Maintenance Stage Can Be Most Difficult

As described earlier, the first major challenge in the change process is to get beyond the stage of denial, and the next major challenge is to stay in the action stage. The third, and for some the most difficult challenge is to move into and stay in the maintenance stage until total termination of the problem habit is realized. Dr. Prochaska reminds us that all stages of change require a series of tasks, a stretch of time in which to try them, and a certain amount of energy and commitment. The action stage typically lasts for several months and there are many opportunities for relapse. Friends and family alike should view these challenges with understanding and compassion because there is a tremendous amount of work involved in successful action.

Maintenance takes all that required work and builds on it. Although it is difficult to accept, forsaking an undesirable behavior may not be enough for some to overcome it for good. Referring back to the mind groove analogy, a lot may depend on just how deep the bad habit groove is. To fully overcome an entrenched bad habit it must be replaced by a new long-term, healthy lifestyle habit.

Prevention Is Still the Best Policy

This realization brings us back full circle to the concept of prevention, where the seven principles of wellness and longevity are critical in preventing any interference with the divine body wisdom. In a very real sense, the maintenance stage offers the opportunity to put one in touch with the Soul or body wisdom by creating and maintaining a mental commitment to a new healthy lifestyle and bodily rhythm, which will eventually lead to permanent termination of whatever bad habits may have existed.

The commitment to a healthy life is one of the very best ways to serve yourself—as well as your family, friends, and humanity in general. Setting an optimum example of wellness and longevity will embody the seven principles of Rite eating, sleeping, thinking, energizing, hydrating, exercising, and embracing a toxin-free lifestyle. Each of these actions should be viewed as a most natural rhythmic way of harmonizing the Soul and physical body for optimum wellness and raising the level of consciousness to happiness and joy, and possible enlightenment during this lifetime.

How to Know Success?

In simple terms, the truth will be self-evident when the person is no longer tempted with the previous addiction. When a person realizes this state, doctors use the academic term "termination," which is the final step in the change process. It will be obvious that the individual is no longer a slave to a bad habit and has most likely followed some version of the above stated change process.

Now armed with the tools for change, come with me to explore the 7 Rite Rules to prepare for physical immortality—and leading a healthy and energetic life in the meantime.

CHAPTER 3
THE RITE RULE #1—DIET
Eat to Live Not Live to Eat

David lounged in one of the chairs in my consultation room, his pale blue eyes sizing me up. "I'm only here because of my wife. Sharon's scared because my doctor says I have diabetes. My parents had it, and they both died young."

I took a look at David's medical tests and could understand Sharon's fears. In addition to high blood-sugar levels, David had high blood pressure and high low-density lipids (LDLs), all of which were life-threatening.

"What am I supposed to do?" he said. "It's just bad genes."

After I questioned David about his lifestyle, however, I was sure his eating habits and sedentary practices were much more to blame for his condition than any genetic predisposition. I was surprised, however, when his body composition test revealed a high level of body fat, 45%, which placed him in a morbidly obese category. Although he was carrying around an extra 30 to 40 pounds, he did not look morbidly obese.

David did not react well to this news. "I don't think my weight is a problem. You should see some of the guys I work with at the plant."

"David," I said, "this isn't about a beauty contest. We're talking about your health. You're only 45 years old. Do you want to live and play with your grandkids, or would you rather let Sharon do that by herself?"

That seemed to shake him up, and he agreed to follow my lifestyle program, which included a food plan free of nearly all man-made products. At the end of a six-month period, David had lost 35 pounds of fat with a drop of body fat percentage to 26%, was down to normal blood sugar and blood pressure, and accomplished all of this without ever having to take prescription drugs. David is now living and eating The Rite Way

Eating properly is the first major rule of the 7 Rite Rules. The word *diet* has no relationship to commonly held images of restricted eating programs associated with weight loss. It is an energy principle that has a major impact on prevention of chronic illnesses. As a clinical nutritionist, I offer specifics on what and how much to eat to optimize wellness and longevity. I often use the rule of hand for how much to eat without having to count calories, as the size of one's hands relates to one's total body mass index. (The rule of hand for proper food volume consumption is discussed later in the chapter.)

In addition to how much to eat, this chapter clearly spells out what specific foods are best and lists them with an emphasis on the benefits of eating the majority of calories from raw natural whole foods. It reviews all of the macro-nutrients such as proteins, fats, fiber, and carbohydrates and how they can best be obtained from organic whole fruits, vegetables, seeds, nuts, and grains. It also emphasizes that all of the micro-nutrients—including vitamins, enzymes, minerals, glyco-proteins, glyco-lipids, flavanoids, and other phyto-nutrients—needed for optimum wellness and longevity are clearly best obtained from raw whole foods containing a wide array of orderly molecular nutrients.

The Rite Diet: Orderly Molecular Energy for the Body

Improper diet is essentially disordered molecular energy and is a major cause of chronic illnesses. (The evils of improper diet are covered more closely in Chapter 7, "The Rite Rule #5—Toxin-Free Living.") However, this chapter starts with the D-R-R-I-T-E-S acronym and the first letter, "D" for Diet. The Rite Diet presents an "ordered molecular energy diet," which is primarily about eating foods that will provide the proper fuel at the cellular level in the form of macro- and micro-nutrients. These nutrients are known to promote vitality and longevity and to help prevent chronic illnesses from occurring by bolstering the immune system and many other bodily functions.

The Rite Diet Rule conjures up a wide spectrum of different images. Some tend to view diet as an eating program that requires restrictions over previous patterns. Others tend to view diet as a temporary eating program that means eating less food until a certain weight objective is obtained. The word "diet" generally evokes a negative feeling with the great majority of the population, but nevertheless a significant number of people seem to be following some type of eating program called a diet most of the time.

In the broadest sense a diet can be healthy or unhealthy depending on the specific foods and quantities included in the program. Diet for purposes of this program means regularly eating the right kinds of foods with proven "ordered molecular nutrients" known to promote long-term vitality, wellness, and longevity. The Rite Diet should be an enjoyable eating process where one regularly pays attention to the quantities and qualities of all foods consumed over their entire life. It does not mean a person has to become a fanatic or obsessive about food ingested. It should be viewed as a process of acquiring knowledge and implementing the wisdom presented here as to which foods are good and which are bad for the body.

Some People Treat Their Cars Better Than Their Bodies

In my lectures, I often use a car analogy to make the point of how important it is to use the right kind of fuel. For example, if the owner's manual clearly states that the driver should use only a premium fuel of 91 octane and the owner pumps gas with an 87 octane into the tank, there are eventually going to be problems. The car may seem to run okay for a tank or two, but serious damage to the fuel injectors and other moving parts will, over time, cause failures to occur. The comparison to the human body involves having the right information about maintaining health, and then taking the right action consistently in order to provide the optimum fuel nutrients for wellness, longevity, and disease prevention.

Unfortunately our bodies do not come with an owner's manual, but the human body isn't that hard to operate and maintain. Many of its systems are automatic and don't require much attention, provided toxins are not interfering with the bodily wisdom. However, as logical and simple as this proposition is, the majority of people are ingesting many toxins in their food, including artificial colorings, preservatives, artificial flavorings, emulsifiers, humectants, antimicrobials, growth hormones, pesticides, parasites, bacteria, virus, molds, and more. Over time, these toxins create chronic negative effects on their wellness and longevity. Most are driven by their emotions and physical desires and many tend to view the consumption of good health promoting foods as needless restrictions to an enjoyable taste-driven lifestyle. In many cases, when the facts about good and bad foods are presented to those who are obsessively taste driven, they simply dismiss or deny the informational truths that may interfere with their present taste-driven eating desires.

Nevertheless, in spite of this condition, the known facts regarding good and bad foods need to be presented for those interested in promoting high vitality, longevity, and prevention of diseases.

What Is the Truth about Healthy Foods?

Getting down to the absolute truths about good foods versus problem foods can be extremely challenging. Many forces with self-serving agendas are at work in the food industry. The food industry is the single largest business sector in America and enormous amounts of dollars are at stake. It is the food processing institutions within this industry that employ a "whatever it takes" marketing strategy to convince the public that they should be consuming their processed products. This situation in many cases contributes to the avalanche of untruths and misinformation that permeates the food processing industry and its markets.

One of the most complete and referenced papers on this issue is presented by Dr. Royal Lee, president of the Nutritional Research Foundation in Milwaukee, Wisconsin. He states, "We have been beset with a follow-the-leader pattern of conduct, led by vicious commercial interests who direct their gullible flock with apparent deliberateness into disastrous pastures to feed on counterfeit foods." His point? It is difficult to convince the people who relish white bread with its dough conditioners, doughnuts made with synthetic grease, and cereals loaded with refined sugars and hydrogenated oils, that there is any connection between these counterfeit foods and their health status. Dr. Lee says that "of course, when a person becomes victimized by arthritis, heart disease, or diabetes, for example, the job of convincing him becomes somewhat easier." Dr. Lee makes the argument that the disregard of nature's basic food laws and the substitution of man-made laws that permit the sale of toxic counterfeit foods to the unprotected public is the number one national health problem. It dwarfs any other health problems caused by drug addiction, alcoholism, smoking, homicides, and auto accidents.

The concerns regarding the truth about quality foods are a major theme presented throughout this chapter. The theme also includes the importance of food quantity and presents the issues of quality and quantity in the form of two sub-rules under The Rite Diet Rule:

- **Diet Sub-Rule A:** Whole natural raw foods contain "ordered molecular energy" and should comprise the major part of all diets for those seeking vibrant wellness, energy, and longevity.
- **Diet Sub-Rule B:** Optimum quantities of whole natural foods should be consumed with a mindset of "eating to live" and not with an attitude of "living to eat."

Quantity: What Are the Facts Regarding How Much to Eat?

Diet sub-rule B deals with the issue of over-consumption. Even good foods can be over-consumed, but this is seldom the case with good natural unprocessed foods. Based on numerous studies, foods that average people overeat tend to be highly processed foods, which are by nature highly synthesized, highly toxic, highly dehydrated, and highly advertised. I have never had a weight loss patient who claimed to be overeating fruits and vegetables. The vast majority of overweight patients reveal that they are primarily addicted to or obsessed over some form of man-made processed foods.

Eat Good Foods In Moderate Amounts

Scientific animal studies and evidence collected within the past twenty years or so convincingly show those animals that eat a minimum of calories live significantly healthier and longer lives. Numerous studies in this area have a high level of repeatability of results and a high level of confidence in the conclusions. While longitudinal studies are still ongoing with humans, it is fair to state that the general consensus among scientists is that a similar correlation to animal studies probably exists.

People who are overweight clearly are prone to increased health problems and live shorter lives, and the heavier they are the less healthy and shorter their lives will be. It may be obvious, but supporting this consensus is the improbability of seeing an obese centenarian. One of the major findings after interviewing many centenarians is that in general they "eat to live" and not "live to eat." They tend to exhibit normal weight and lifestyles of moderation in most endeavors.

Overeating: The Dominant Variable

In the discussion of overeating and the connection to overweight conditions, it is obvious that there is more than one variable at work in the total body mass equation. Food energy input is one variable and energy output is another major variable. (There are some who believe in other variables such as heredity, but as you'll see later in the chapter, the evidence doesn't always support it.)

Although the body consumes or expends energy even while resting, it certainly outputs more when the body is active in the form of regular and sustained body movements. But, if a weight management physician was forced to supply an answer as to which variable is dominant in weight control, most would come down on the side of over-consumption in that few people burn more calories than they consume in today's environment. Many credible studies support this latter position.

The Best Foods Contain "Ordered Molecular Energy"

There probably is no perfect diet that is optimum for everybody. The variables that make for an optimum diet are numerous and may include such aspects as age, gender, genetics, blood type, ethnic background, resting metabolic rate, level of activity, and even hot or cold environment.

The Rite Diet Rule is exceedingly simple and easy to follow and is based on supplying the body with optimum "ordered molecular energy," or OME, with an absence of toxic elements. The concept of OME simply means that the molecules within the foods consumed are filled with orderly non-radical, non-toxic atoms. An orderly atom is an atom that has all of its electrons matching the total number of protons. A disorderly atom is one that has fewer electrons than protons. Atoms with these extra protons are generally referred to as free radicals and can be destructive to the body at the cellular level. They steal electrons from atoms in healthy cells and start chain reactions that often lead to disruption of cell function and/or death of the cell.

The initial formation of a free radical can occur when chemicals, heat, air, pressure, or combinations thereof are applied to foods, causing them to lose electrons. For example, when an apple is cut open and the insides are exposed to air, it begins to oxidize (lose electrons) and turn brown as the atoms on the surface become free radicals.

It is with this "orderly molecular energy" or OME concept in mind that I made diet sub-rule A about eating primarily whole foods.

Whole foods means primarily fruits, vegetables, seeds, grains, nuts, legumes, herbs, spices, and selected seafoods. Eating these foods will supply OME in macro- and micro-nutrient forms of protein, fats, fiber, and carbohydrates necessary to maintain proper energy and lean body mass. These nutritious food groups will also build the immune system, promote proper digestion and elimination, supply nutrition for proper brain functioning, and for the most part support the vital endocrine glandular system. A listing of these foods is presented at the end of this chapter. A listing is also shown on a sliding scale for foods that are less than optimum.

Less Than Optimum Foods

Animal products, such as meat, fish, and dairy, can be consumed but there is almost always the risk of heavy contamination and toxins of some sort ranging from parasites and bacteria to heavy metals, synthetic hormones, antibiotics, and pesticides. Some processed foods can also be consumed, but here again there is nearly always a large toxicity concern. A list of animal and processed foods is shown later, but they are relegated to lower levels where there are increased risks of toxins and disordered molecular energy created during cooking.

Some Processed Foods May Be Okay

I highly recommend that all processed foods that you buy in packages, boxes, jars, or cans be labeled "organic" and "kosher." When a product is labeled kosher, the consumer can know that responsible independent inspectors (in the form of Jewish Rabbis) have initially scrutinized the facility where they are made. These inspectors also return more often to ensure that sanitary conditions are being maintained in order to warrant the kosher label. Generally, products labeled kosher carry stricter standards and offer more reliability than those only inspected by the government.

Buying Organic

With products labeled as organic, the consumer can be reasonably assured that they are free of pesticides, herbicides, hormones, and antibiotics. Freedom from these contaminants (as stated in the Rite Toxin-free Rule) is crucial to wellness, energy, and longevity, and is a critical component for the effectiveness of all 7 Rite Rules. (See Chapter 7, "The Rite Rule #5—Toxin-Free Living" for further discussion on various levels of organic assurance and for more specifics on toxic foods.)

Although contamination concerns exist regarding natural unprocessed foods, it is nowhere near the level assigned to animal and processed foods. A rule to follow before purchasing natural foods is to look for "organic" identification in the form of a label or sign on or above the produce food sections. Organic identification means that the growers have pledged no pesticides, no biotechnology, no sewer-sludge or synthetic fertilizers, and no irradiation methods have been used in the production of their organic foods. While these natural foods may cost a little more, it ensures that your body will not have to process those entities that are known to be toxic.

Finding the Best Whole Foods

Under ideal conditions, the very best way to consume natural raw foods would be to pick them directly from your own garden and wash and eat them the same day. Here you would know that contaminants are at a minimum, handling and storage processes have not deteriorated, and no other contaminants have been added such as bacteria and mold. Since growing all your own food is pretty unrealistic for the vast majority of the population, you should at least know how and where your food gets to market. You should know that all natural products are handled at least twice before you select them from the supermarket produce section: the first time by hand from a picker in the field, and at least one more time by the supermarket employee placing them in the produce section. Who knows how many customers may have handled the produce before you finally select those to bring home?

Lest you think I'm giving too much attention to contaminants and possible toxins, you should realize that these entities can cause serious problems, particularly in people with compromised immune systems. Even with an optimum immune system, it is likely some bodily function will become compromised with a constant ingestion of toxins from additives such as artificial flavorings and growth hormones to bacteria and pesticides. Regular intake of high levels of toxins can lead to deterioration of even the best of livers, kidneys, intestines, and lymphatic and immune systems.

Little Parasites, Molds, and Microbes Create Big Problems

Beyond these concerns are the pesky bacterial, parasitic, and mold problems that may be present depending on storage and handling techniques. However, as a general precaution the following steps should be taken before consuming raw foods:

- All fruits, vegetables, and legumes, where the skin or outer covering is to be consumed, should be washed thoroughly and sprayed with lemon juice or diluted grapefruit seed extract. This cleansing process is particularly important with any root foods, such as carrots, that will be consumed raw. If any dirt is left and consumed the risk of bacterial and or parasitic infection is high.
- All raw seeds and nuts should be sprinkled with powdered vitamin C. The major risk with seeds and nuts has to do with mold that can accumulate during storage.

> *"A good scare is worth more to a man than good advice."*
>
> —Edgar Watson Howe

How Much and What Is Optimum to Eat?

As stated earlier, minimizing food intake has been clearly shown to correlate with optimum health and longevity... but what is minimum? Many variables should be considered when determining what is best to eat. And it's not just about how much food you should eat, but how much of the best foods should you eat.

The Rule of Hand May Be the Best Guide for Consumption

People who care about what they put in their bodies—who eat organic and raw whole foods—tend to be a more normal weight because they focus on "eating to live" and eating the right foods, not just eating only for pleasure with processed, overly sugared, overly toxin-filled foods, overly cooked foods that others may want to gorge themselves on.

Some of the variables associated with optimum volume of foods have to do with height and weight, gender, age, activity, and metabolism. Therefore, it is inappropriate to try and specify the amount of food in weight or calories that is right for everyone. I have found that generally, the "rule of hand" works best—as the hands are coupled in the form of a bowl, a heaping bowl of vegetables and a heaping bowl of fruits should be consumed daily. Since the hands are generally in the right proportion to height and weight, this rule seems to work for the vast majority. Generally, I'd advocate people consuming their many colored vegetables in the form of a salad with a healthy dressing. Additionally, a person should eat slowly because raw vegetables should be enjoyed and savored with a ritual of proper chewing to ensure oral enzyme saturation. I recommend somewhere between 21 and 50 chews per mouthful. In other words, whatever number of chews it takes to get the food to a near liquid level should be done before swallowing.

Vegetables Should Be Dressed Up!

According to my taste buds, vegetables are delicious, but not everyone feels the same way. People who are not accustomed to eating raw vegetables often have difficulty eating a heaping bowl daily. This is where dressing up veggies can present a whole new avenue for food enjoyment for some people. To the extent that they can be dressed up with herbs and good oils and spices, they will become more palatable and desirable. Many who shunned vegetables before will actually look forward to consuming these health promoting foods on a daily basis.

The optimum dressing includes half of a fresh squeezed lemon and a combination of linseed, flax seed, borage, and/or hemp oil. For a large salad, 1 to 2 tablespoons of dressing should be enough. You can use organic vinegar in place of lemon juice, but there is the risk of mold contamination. Olive oil is acceptable on occasions but it lacks the omega 3 and 6 nutrient values and is primarily an omega 9 fat. It is the omega 3 and 6 fats, in equal balance, that are absolutely essential in the diet in order to maintain proper body and brain functioning. When consuming these nutrients in oil form, it is very important to use only opaque containers, and after opening the container it should be refrigerated. (Light, heat, and air are known to deteriorate oils. Exposure to these elements result in free radicals, rancid oil, and twisted trans molecules.)

In addition to lemon juice and nutritious oils for salads, you can also add walnuts, legumes such as garbanzo beans, celery seeds, sunflower seeds, flax seeds, and herbs and seasonings like onions, garlic, ginger root, basil, thyme, coriander, and fenugreek. Rotate these in moderate amounts in each salad.

Fruits and Vegetables: The Natural Medicine Chest

In addition to the vital nutrients you'll get from your daily dose of vegetables, also be aware that these wonderful foods, living in the storage bin of your refrigerator, are a powerful medicine chest. In this chest, you will unlock natural hydrated major nutrients for illness prevention and cure. One of the major reasons raw fruits and vegetables are so effective in preventing chronic illnesses is that they contain essential nutrients in the form of carbohydrates, vitamins, enzymes, anti-oxidants, and minerals in a hydrated environment. Ample amounts of water, with trace minerals within the plant, sets up effective digestion in the intestines and provides optimum absorption by the cells and micro-nutrients needed for proper cell mitochondria, golgi, and endoplasmic reticulum functioning. The nutrients and cell parts listed here are not complete. There are many more nutrients—including sugars such as xylose, galactose, glucose, mannose, N-acetylgalactosamine—which can link up and form more than 1,000 different trisaccharides. There are many proteins and enzymes, such as lectins, glycans, amino acids, and glycoconjugates, that result in gene transcription factors producing molecules that serve as helpful cell messengers. These findings are examples of fast-paced developments under the new science of Nutrigenomics, which tells us more about how micro-nutrients affect cellular and bodily health. However, all you really have to know is that a daily bowl full of multi-colored, raw, fresh, organic fruits and vegetables will play a major role in keeping you healthy with the macro inputs of ordered molecular energy.

Nuts and Seeds Provide Clean Fat and Protein

One handful of seeds and nuts each should be consumed daily. A handful is defined as the amount that can be held in one hand with the fingers semicurled into a position where the tips of the fingers are about two inches from the base of the palm.

Raw nuts and seeds are nutritious foods but are grossly under-consumed by the general population. These natural foods should be given much more attention as an effective way for absorbing good protein and essential fatty acids. Instead of reaching for processed snacks such as potato chips, pretzels, crackers, and the like, seeds and nuts would be a much better choice because these natural foods contain good fats and proteins without the downside presented by simple carbohydrates and toxins contained in processed snacks.

Virtually all seeds and nuts are healthy to consume, and the more variety the better. A listing of seeds includes flax, safflower, sesame, pumpkin, and sunflower. A listing of nuts includes almond, brazil, cashew, chestnut, coconut, filbert, hazelnut, macadamia, peanut, pecan, pinenut, pistachio, and walnut. These seeds and nuts should be rotated throughout your diet as much as possible because they each contain various amounts of healthy fats, protein, and minerals. (Walnuts should be given extra attention because they naturally provide the omega 3 essential fatty acids in which many people are deficient.)

Whole Grains Provide Complex Carbs, Fat, and Protein

Grains should be consumed on a one-handful-a-day basis. The volume of grains should be measured in their raw state with a total volume that will not exceed a handful—measured the same way as you would measure seeds and nuts. The very best way to eat grains is in their whole kernel state, as described later in this chapter.

Refined Grains Are Problem Foods

Whole grains provide many wonderful nutrients in the form of vitamins, minerals, fiber, carbohydrates, and proteins and should become a regular part of everyone's daily diet.

The major problem with grains has to do with refined grains. They furnish the base from which simple carbo-*dehydrated* products are built. Anchoring this point in your mind is very important because many food manufacturers sell large amounts of processed grains to the public each year in the form of cereals, cookies, cakes, donuts, crackers, and chips. These types of simple "carbo-*dehydrated*" foods contribute substantially to our many national health problems. These products are also responsible for the growing obesity epidemic in our adults and children. Refined grains have the fiber and other nutrients processed out, making the once nutritional hydrated grain into a simple "carbo-*dehydrate*." In this form it becomes a refined starch, which when consumed causes a quick conversion to sugar and a resultant conversion to fat in the body. When you consume whole grains in the form of whole oats, barley, wheat, and rice with all the natural fats, proteins, fiber, and carbohydrates held together in a natural state, this problem is virtually eliminated.

When one examines and ponders the contents of a whole kernel of wheat, it becomes obvious that nature has provided a marvelous encapsulated and protected package of fats, protein, and fiber carbohydrated nutrients. After soaking in water for several hours these grains become some of the best forms of nutritious edible foods. You can top them off with cut-up fruit, sprinkle with walnuts and cinnamon, and you have a tasty and enjoyable way to start off the day with a well-balanced breakfast.

So, why would an informed person want to eat boxed cereal grains that have lost the protection of the outer shell and nutrients and are now exposed to the risk of mold during storage? Moreover, grains purchased as cereal have survived a refining process where most nutrients are removed and refined sugars are added to entice people with a hyper-sweetened taste. Grain processors even add a toxin-filled synthetic to create a crispy texture in the form of processed hydrogenated oils. (There are a few boxed cereals that are considered acceptable and are produced from sprouted grains.)

Proteins, Fats, and Carbohydrates in the Natural Ratios

For the past few years, America's attention has been focused on diet—and the optimum combination of macro-nutrients such as protein, fat, and carbohydrates. For example, some diets advocate certain proportions such as 30% fat, 30% protein, and 40% carbohydrates, whereas others favor large amounts of animal fat and protein and small amounts of carbohydrates. Many diet recommendations fall somewhere in between. What most of these diets overlook is that while all natural foods contain some percentage of protein, too many people seriously over-consume protein when they focus solely on meat and dairy. Over-consumption of animal protein is a serious matter and can be associated with osteoporosis, arthritis, and heart disease.

In addition to undervaluing protein in plant products, these diets also often overlook the amount of essential fats contained in natural foods. Animal products and processed oils are not necessary to get the proper amount of fat into the diet.

All Fats Aren't Bad

The fats present in natural foods such as nuts, seeds, fruits, vegetables, grains, and legumes are healthy fats and should be consumed daily according to the hand rule. Many seeds and nuts have high amounts of omega fatty acids, some reaching close to 80 percent of total calories in each unit, and should be consumed on a regular basis. This includes fruits such as avocados and coconuts, and even though they have a high saturated fat content, their medium chain fatty acids offer many health promoting attributes. These fruits should be factored into the "rule of hand" volume along with seeds and nuts. (For example, if a handful of nuts or seeds have been consumed, avocados and/or coconuts should not be consumed that day.) Tofu and soybeans should be included in this equation as well because they contain up to 49 percent saturated fat with high amounts of medium chain fatty acids.

70-15-15—Nature's Ratio

It is interesting to note that by consuming natural whole foods using the hand rule, all of the macro-nutrients of protein, fat, fiber, and carbohydrates will represent approximately the following ratios: 15% protein, 15% fat, and 70% fiber and carbohydrates. An optimized healthy body is generally composed of nearly 70% water, 15 % protein, and 15% fat by weight. Many complex carbohydrates (such as fruit) are approximately 70% water, 15% fat, and 15% protein by weight. Although there are some variances it is clear that the 70-15-15 ratio appears in nature quite often. If you're serious about following a diet for optimized wellness and longevity, this ratio can be used as a standard to be followed for good health.

There are negative effects of over-consuming marginal fats and protein. The 30-40-30 diet popular in some books today should be reevaluated before it becomes a part of your regular lifestyle. Additionally, diets that advocate extremely low intake of carbohydrates replaced with lots of protein should be avoided because they cause the body to produce large quantities of ketones. While the idea is that ketones break down unusable fat, much of the weight loss dieters see on these plans comes from water expelled to rid the body of the poisonous ketones.

I have yet to meet a patient who claims to be overeating raw fruits or vegetables. The body's wisdom seems to know it has had enough good calories. However, chemicals and some natural components of processed foods and animal products short-circuit or blind the body's physiological wisdom, making it too easy to over-consume these foods. (Yet another reason why today's artificially produced fat substitutes or oils produced by hydrogenation processes are harmful. They mask the body's natural ability to register satisfaction and cause you to overeat without even realizing it.)

Food Tables

The following table rates a variety of foods as to their nutrient density of vitamins, minerals, fiber, protein, complex carbohydrates, and healthy fats.

Best Foods

oranges	coconuts	wheat germ
limes	pineapple	beets
tangerines	apples	peas
bananas	pears	celery
strawberries	watermelon	radicchio
cantaloupe	crenshaw-leeks	red cabbage
apricots	sunflower seeds	pumpkin seeds
papaya	chard	barley
cherries	pumpkin	wheat
avocados	brussels	oats
blueberries	sprouts	millet
grapes	tomatoes	amaranth
honeydew	winter squash	spirulina
melon	kale	rye
plums	parsley	brown rice
rhubarb	asparagus	lima beans
grapefruits	potatoes	corn
peaches, melons	radishes	brown beans
parsley pasta*	zucchini	pop corn
spinach pasta*	kidney beans	flax oil
beet greens	garbanzo beans	borage oil
cauliflower	yams	sesame oil
lettuce	turnips	flax seeds
dandelion	navy beans	walnuts
greens	garlic	almonds
endive	green peppers	halibut*
spinach	carrots	sole*
sprouts	black-eyed peas	cod*
onions	pinto beans	tuna*
cabbage	soy beans	salmon*

Fair Foods

prunes	raisins	dates	peanuts turkey*
granola	dried fruits	whole grain pasta*	
chicken*	meats*	eggs	

Poor Foods

molasses	pancakes	most cheeses	most pies, clams
waffles	white rice	cookies, cake	
canned fruits	oysters	milk	ice cream
crackers, pizza	white pasta	shrimp	white flour
lobster	margarine	organ meats	
creamed vegetables	canned vegetables		

Bad Foods

sausage	sugar	all soft drinks	mayonnaise	
ketchup	syrups	jams	butter	
bacon	coffee	all alcoholic drinks	chips	potato
chips	pretzels	hot dogs	tea	most
spices	gelatin desserts	Tabasco	salad	
dressings	salami	pastries	doughnuts	
soup mixes	pickles	lard		
sugared cereals	hydrogenated fats and oils			
most packaged foods				
all products with sugar and preservatives				

*These foods require cooking and although rated as good to fair because of their macro-nutrients, depending on temperatures and length of cooking, they are at risk for creating disorganized energies and the adverse consequences that come from disordered energies.

Good Food Is the Best Medicine

Generally speaking, if you follow the 7 Rite Rules contained in this book you should have little need for commercial medicines or other types of nutritional supplementation. Eating a well-balanced, whole raw food diet as described in this chapter is an important first sub- rule. However, if you have been diagnosed with one or more illnesses described in the

Introduction, you may need temporary supplementation primarily to cover deficient nutrient and / or toxic conditions.

As a general rule I prefer to see the test results of nutritional laboratory testing with hair, saliva, stool, urine, or blood samples before supplements or cleansing programs are recommended. For example, if the test results indicate a need, I can recommend supplementation directed to reduce the aging effects of free radicals to optimize wellness, energy, and longevity. Reducing free radicals becomes particularly important the older one gets. I generally recommend testing for supplementation needs (including basic anti-oxidants to reduce free radicals), at around the age of 50 or if patients have symptoms indicating a prevalent lack of certain nutrients (literally modern malnutrition.)

Some of the more popular anti-oxidants include vitamins A, C, and E. Additional anti-oxidants like CoQ10, alpha lipoic acid, n-acetyl carnitine, bioflavonoids, isoflavonoids, catechins, proanthocyanidins, and pycnogenols can also be considered as possible supplementation to reduce or minimize the effects of free radicals. The subject of proper supplementation is too broad to be adequately covered in this book, let alone one chapter. Remember that prevention of disease is the keystone of the 7 Rite Rules and if you eat the recommended foods and follow my eating plan, you should see minimal appearance of free radicals, generally minimizing the need for supplementation. Nevertheless, the appendix has a listing of laboratory tests that I recommend before most supplementation programs are started.

Buyer Beware of Faulty Supplements

The issues of quality and effectiveness are a major concern whenever supplements are discussed. Many supplements on the market today not only lack quality, but also present serious health risks. The entire supplement industry should be viewed as a buyer-beware environment. Not that government regulation solves all problems, but supplements are not held to high consistency, quality, or manufacturing standards and can vary greatly in composition, potency, and quality from maker to maker. I have personally tested many over-the-counter supplements for toxins analyzing for chemical make-up and found over 90 percent of the supplements tested have various levels of toxins. Some of the most prevalent toxins found in the most popular vitamins and minerals included heavy metals, lanthanides, thulium, isopropyl alcohol, benzene, decane, hexanes, and other chemicals. My suspicion is that many of these toxins become a part of the product as a result of faulty equipment cleaning practices employed in the production of the supplement capsules and tablets. In addition many of the gelatin capsules tested contained inherent harmful properties because of animal origins.

Beyond the issue of toxicity there is the question of how much of the supplement is actually absorbed into the body. With supplements in tablet form, studies have shown less than 5 percent of the advertised nutrients actually get absorbed because the binders that hold the tablets together do not break down properly in most digestive systems.

Because of these problems and other issues associated with supplementation, I highly recommend you purchase supplements only from knowledgeable and caring health practitioners. Caring practitioners are those who place illness prevention and health restoration as high priorities for their patients. If a patient requires supplements, they should be of proven high quality and effectiveness. I'd also caution against health practitioners who dispense supplements through network or multi-level marketing organizations because their priorities and values may be more directed toward profits rather than your welfare. Before committing to a consultation with a health practitioner, ask if any multi-level product supplements are used in the practice. If the answer is yes, just be aware that the doctor's priorities might be directed toward building a multi-level money-making organization.

If you suffer from any chronic health issues (see list of diseases in the Introduction) that you deem need a doctor's assistance, you should seek out health practitioners with a background and training in nutrition and who dispense products distributed exclusively for health practitioners.

Eating The Rite Way Is Worth It

One final thought regarding the subject of putting the Rite foods into your body. Many people, including many of my patients, have remarked on the nerdy images associated with health freaks, or "rabbit food eaters." "I have to have something that sticks to my ribs" and "I need to feel full" are remarks I often hear. Or how about this one? "I'd rather be dead than to give up ice cream, or french fries, or cakes, or cookies, or pies, or candy, or jams, or soda pop...."

If you are feeling this way, I challenge you to visit an assisted care facility in your area. I have visited many around the country and I've come to see a typical scene: Dozens, and in many facilities hundreds, of elderly residents line the hallways in wheelchairs and in beds, many in pain with an inability to keep their heads up straight or speak clearly. Most are victims of heart attacks, strokes, cancer, and diabetes, and cannot care for themselves. They can't eat or go to the bathroom on their own. They need constant care, and in some cases are near vegetable status. And they're not getting better. They are only deteriorating.

The tragedy is that virtually all of the misery and hardship I've seen is preventable—I firmly believe—with a healthy diet and lifestyle. Think about your future and view this first rule as a major step toward preparing you for the prospects of immortality. As you read through the rest of the book, you'll see that the 7 Rite Rules, compared to the negative alternatives, are simple and easy to follow.

Resveratrol: proven to help retard aging

Here is an exception for skepticism regarding multilevel products.

Resveratrol was made popular as a result of the French Paradox studies that proved even though the French were known to eat diets filled with many fats and other negative ingredients they had fewer cardio vascular problems and lived longer than many other nationalities. The major reason for reduced heart disease was attributed to the ingestion of Resveratrol found in the skin of red grapes and preserved from air and light oxidation in the corked bottles of red wine. After these studies the search was on to capture Resveratrol in air and light tight containers and ingest it without the negative effects of alcohol. Today Resveratrol mainly comes from the roots of a Japanese plant and in cocoa beans which exist in potent form within some dark chocolates.

Resveratrol is sold in many forms including liquids, tablets, capsules and powder. However, aside from grape skins, Japanese plant root and chocolate it is only highly potent when processed in supplement form if it is sealed in light and air tight capsules. Resvantage is a multi level company that has spent many years looking for a practical way to package the product in a light and air tight capsule, and recently they found success and patented a capsule with Pfizer Inc. performing the encapsulation.

Resveratrol is available from Resvantage via tel: 949-689-4465 Resveratrol is also contained in my private brand sugar free chocolate bar labeled "Dr. Rite's Sugar Free Chocolate withResveratrol" The chocolate bars can be found at most health food stores.

CHAPTER 4

THE RITE RULE #2—REST

Proper Rest Is Crucial for Wellness

When Rick, a 34-year-old stockbroker and self-professed entrepreneur, came to see me, he asked if I could supply him with a pill to compensate for his lack of sleep and symptoms of fatigue, anxiety, depression, and chest pains. The consultation revealed that during the last nine months he had gotten involved in several other businesses requiring at least eight to ten hours of work a day, including weekends.

He claimed that getting up at 4:30 a.m. was necessary to satisfy his brokerage clients and that although he was getting less than six hours of restless sleep a night, he was sure that some type of supplement must be available to help overcome his symptoms. Rick was a typical "type A personality," exuding confidence, seemingly believing he was invincible, and that there wasn't a situation he couldn't handle. In fact, he boasted several times "I really don't need much sleep."

Rick needed some clear advice to help resolve some of his conflicting health views. I told him point blank, "Your body needs more sleep in order to properly repair damage done during the day." I also advised him to reduce his business activities to a point where he could wake up without an alarm clock. "This will tell you how much sleep your body needs." I let him know that if he didn't get more rest he was likely headed for increased illness symptoms. I counseled him on promoting the flow of the master sleep hormone melatonin by following all of the wellness and longevity rules, and of course in his case I emphasized following the Rite Rest Rule. I told him to call me if his symptoms didn't disappear after a month or so of sufficient sleep.

Rick called about 30 days later and expressed amazement over how much difference one additional hour of sleep made in his overall "well-being." He wondered why none of the other doctors, who performed many expensive diagnostic tests, never emphasized that a lack of sleep could be a major cause of his symptoms. Rick is now sleeping and living The Rite Way.

I suppose one could argue that Rick should have been able to figure out the cause of his problems on his own. The principle may seem so obvious a requirement for health that little if anything needs to be said. However, research has shown millions suffer from illnesses caused by insufficient rest. In this chapter, I'll tell you why everyone must determine their unique need for proper sleep and how to do it. I define the amount of proper rest as the amount necessary for you to achieve a state of well-being.

The "R" in the D-R-R-I-T-E-S acronym represents Rite Rule #2—Rest. The Rite Rest is the form of sleep that will promote daily well-being and wellness over the long run.

Getting By with Minimum Sleep Can Be a Problem

Some people seem to think that getting by on little sleep is a sign of superhuman ability and worth bragging about. They tend to believe that more waking hours translate into more hours for work activity. What these people don't realize is that they must eventually pay for lack of sleep in some way.

According to a National Sleep Foundation poll, at least two-thirds of adults say concentrating and handling stress on the job is more difficult when they are sleepy. More than half say that decision making and problem solving are more difficult, and that the quantity and quality of their work is diminished when they are sleepy.

Some believe that people will naturally sleep when they are tired, but studies have shown that people need to follow a certain rhythm or pattern in order to facilitate proper rest. Sleep is necessary for the body to repair itself and rebuild at the cellular level.

However, in today's culture many challenges make it difficult to adhere to this basic wisdom. Nevertheless, this chapter reviews the basic need for rest and presents the dysfunctional consequences that result from not properly satisfying the body's need for rest. In addition, I'll offer some suggestions for helping you achieve the necessary amount of sleep for health and well-being. I define well-being in this case as a state that includes general physical health but with more emphasis on mental awareness and alertness, which promotes problem solving and decision making and also generally creates a sense of wanting to be active and involved.

Rhythmic Rest Is Needed for Bodily Maintenance

Fundamental well-being is promoted with proper rejuvenation and rebuilding of brain and body cellular structures. Your body's cellular structures repair themselves during sleep. This process is so critical that virtually every chronic disease can have as a foundational cause a lack of sufficient sleep, and in order for lasting healing to occur your body must obtain sufficient sleep. Moreover, replenishment of neurotransmitters (chemical messengers in the brain like dopamine, norepinephrine, and serotonin) occur only during the deepest sleep phases. These phases have been documented to occur for only about 45 minutes per four hours of sleep for most people. Ideally it should occur twice during a good night's sleep. It is important to realize that these deep phases of sleep may not occur in the presence of artificial stimulants, artificial sedation, or excessive stress. The deep phases may also be impaired if there is a severe nutritional deficiency of essential amino acids or by poor eating habits (say just before bed) or consumption of alcohol. These amino acids are precursors necessary for producing sufficient neurotransmitters to induce deep sleep states.

Follow Your Unique Need for Sleep

While there is a wide range of time required for each individual to achieve proper rejuvenation and cellular rebuilding, most everyone really knows their own unique amount of sleep time required for them to feel good or have a sense of well-being. When you realize your own personal time requirement, you should give it a priority in your lifestyle to ensure that the amount of sleep needed for your well-being is achieved.

One of the most accurate ways to determine the amount of sleep necessary is to fall asleep without any supplements and to wake up feeling well rested naturally without an alarm clock. This should be done over several nights with notes taken to remind yourself as to the amount of time necessary for a healthy night's sleep. This finding should then be incorporated into a rhythmic lifestyle that will put you to bed at a time that allows you to awake at a required time without an alarm. This advice may seem impractical to some who must be at work at a specific time and therefore believe an alarm clock is necessary to ensure waking up on time. To this concern I offer the same advice I give to many patients: Once you have established your unique need for X hours of sleep, you must fulfill this unique need by making it a priority requirement in your lifestyle and retire at a time that will ensure natural compliance.

Lack of Sleep Affects All the Rite Rules

It should be obvious to most people that not getting the right amount of sleep will adversely impact their behavior. If you're not getting enough sleep, it's going to be a challenge for you to follow the other Rite Rules for wellness. Lack of sleep can disrupt eating and exercise patterns, making it easy to skip exercise and eat a poor diet. It makes it difficult to drink the right amount of water and set aside time to restore the body's energy flow and balance. And lastly, insufficient rest will adversely impact the detoxification process as a result of eating time-saving, convenient, packaged foods.

You Owe It to Your Body to Establish a Rest Rhythm

If you are not getting enough sleep because of time commitments to work, family, friends, or otherwise, you owe it to yourself and the people around you to make a change immediately. For all of the health reasons stated above, a change should be viewed as imperative and given a priority. If the lack of sleep is due to the inability to fall asleep or to a pattern of waking and not being able to fall back to sleep, some of the following suggestions may prove helpful.

Some Suggestions for Sleep Disorders

The pineal gland secretes melatonin. Melatonin is a major hormone that performs as an anti-oxidant, immune system builder, mood elevator, and sleep inducer. It is considered to be the closest substance we have to a natural sleeping pill. Its release is almost entirely confined to the nighttime, and the amount of melatonin we produce and have available for storage is directly related to how much deep sleep we get. For example, elderly people with insomnia have been found to have half the amount of melatonin stored in their body compared to young people.

Here we are presented with an apparent dilemma: Melatonin is produced and stored during the sleeping state, but if a lack of melatonin is caused by insufficient sleep, the body's ability to produce enough melatonin is impaired, which can also contribute to further sleep disorders.

Fortunately, several steps can be employed to correct this condition. Taking a melatonin supplement may help many people start to get sufficient deep sleep, which will then provide the conditions for naturally producing melatonin. If it's working, a melatonin supplement should not be necessary for extended periods. As a matter of fact, the supplement should be viewed as a kick-start procedure, because sustained usage will likely send a message to the pineal gland to stop producing this wonderful hormone.

For most people, somewhere between 1 and 3 milligrams of a melatonin supplement just before bedtime is normally sufficient over a three-night period. However, even though this supplement is available over the counter, your doctor should be consulted for a specific dosage suitable for your body make-up and particular sleeping disorder, as well as for a reputable brand.

A natural way to promote the flow of melatonin is to eat three or four leafs of lettuce about 20 minutes before bedtime. Although I generally do not advocate eating before bedtime, the benefits of the amino acid tryptophan, which is contained in every molecule of lettuce, acts directly to induce the flow of melatonin and should produce a need to sleep.

Regular Exercise Can Be Best for Inducing Sleep

An even more desirable method of stimulating the secretion of the melatonin hormone is through the increased production of natural growth hormone. Natural growth hormone can serve to stimulate the flow of melatonin, and one of the best ways to help ensure the proper amounts of growth hormone is through regular and sustained anaerobic exercises. In addition to an anaerobic resistance exercise routine, performed earlier in the day, you should also take a regular supplementation of 2–5 grams of amino acids such as L arginine and L glutamine an hour or so before bedtime. The effect of these routines on promoting growth hormone can be dramatic during sleep. I believe the process of exercise in and of itself will help the body naturally induce sleep, and several studies have shown that anaerobic exercise during the day coupled with the aforementioned amino acids at night have been highly effective in producing growth hormone, with the amino acids acting as a precursor to stimulating the flow of melatonin. (For more on recommended anaerobic exercises, see Chapter 8, "The Rite Rule #6—Exercise.")

On average, most people require 7–8 hours of sleep each night. Older people may require less and infants more. Persons experiencing persistent fatigue despite getting 7–8 hours of sleep are likely to be suffering from underlying metabolic and/or nutrient deficiencies. If this sounds familiar you should consider being tested for toxic conditions and/or nutrient deficiencies. (See the appendix for information on how to get these tests done.)

Some Additional Tips for Problem Sleepers

If you're still having problems sleeping, follow these guidelines to check for other possible contributing factors:

- Your bedroom should be viewed as a sanctuary for sleep.
- In order to get solid, uninterrupted sleep, the room should be blackened with dark drapes or eyeshades should be used to maintain darkness after the sun has come up.
- The bedroom should have no television or radio. Many people have developed a habit of watching the late evening news or late-night talk shows. If these shows are impinging on your time to fall asleep and wake up naturally without an alarm clock, they must be avoided.
- Also, if you fall asleep while the television is on, the light from the TV will interfere with proper sleep and the production of melatonin, along with all the attendant problems that creates.
- No food should be consumed for at least two hours before bedtime.
- No liquids should be consumed for at least an hour before bedtime. (The preceding two tips are important but can be deviated from if you want to eat several leafs of lettuce 20 minutes before bedtime to promote tryptophan production.)
- If you have to get up during the night to use the bathroom, use a red night light. A white night light or overhead light may curtail the production of melatonin.
- No electronic devices should be connected to the bed (such as electric blankets and heating pads). All electronics create an electric field that will interfere with the cellular repair process that occurs during deep sleep.

- If you find yourself troubled with the day's events or are preoccupied with pressing problems, it is often helpful to commit these concerns to paper before bedtime so you can forget they exist until the next day. Keep a notepad and pen on the bedside table. You can then wake up the next morning with a clear mind and a fresh approach to your problems.
- Finally, you may want to employ a form of self-hypnosis after your head hits the pillow by simply repeating a mantra such as "I'm going to sleep, I'm going to sleep, I'm going to sleep, I love sleeping, I love sleeping."

Daytime Rest and Relaxation

Beyond the physical benefits of sufficient nighttime sleep, it is important to realize that there are benefits from proper resting and relaxation practices that may be used during the day. A simple 10–15 minutes of quiet time after lunch can work wonders in restoring energy levels and in helping to cope with stress. In addition it might be helpful to plan on another 10–15 minutes of quiet time in the middle of the afternoon.

Meditation Can Be Used as a Restful Technique

Meditation can be performed during any quiet time. This regular routine of mental stillness to quiet the mind often helps to reduce stress and promote a relaxed feeling.

There are many forms of meditation, some of which focus on raising consciousness and are intended to increase spiritual awareness, but there are also several other forms with simple relaxation as the aim. The key point in simple meditation for relaxation is to strive for stilling the mind by bringing your attention to the middle of your forehead between the eyebrows. A mantra or prayer can be employed to help facilitate stilling the mind. A mantra many people find effective is to simply repeat the musical scale with the traditional solfege syllables Do, Re, Mi, Fa, Sol, La, Ti, Do. Any prayer or affirmation that you have memorized can also serve to still the mind and help you relax and relieve stress.

Meditation may not physiologically make up for a regular lack of sleep, but it has been shown to help people cope and to help reduce stress.

Stilling the Mind Requires Practice

Stilling the mind can be a challenging endeavor. Some claim the effort is comparable to trying to stop a monkey from jumping around from tree to tree. Like most exercises, meditation requires practice in order to get good results, and most people who intently focus on stilling the mind eventually experience a satisfying difference.

Many books, videos, and audiotapes are available at most bookstores for teaching relaxation and stress reduction, and many communities also offer classes on how to effectively relax through meditation exercises.

Take the Rest and Sleep Test

As an aid to determining whether or not you need more sleep, some experts measure your degree of daytime sleepiness based on the following scale.

How likely are you to fall asleep during the following situations? Give yourself a score based on 0=never doze, 1=slight chance, 2=moderate chance, 3=high chance.

TEST FOR SLEEP DEPRIVATION

- Sitting and reading
- Watching TV
- Sitting inactive in a public place such as theater or meeting
- As a passenger in a car for an hour without a break
- Lying down to rest in the afternoon
- Sitting and talking to someone
- Sitting quietly after lunch (not having had any alcohol)
- In a car stopped in traffic

Now add up your scores. If you scored more than 10, you may have heavy to extreme sleep debt, and you should use the methods described in this chapter to correct the condition.

The Rite Rest Rule is clearly important and should become a priority in developing a rhythmic lifestyle along with all of the other rules. This rule will serve you well in helping to maintain a state of wellness, high energy, and longevity, and further open up the prospects for achieving immortality.

CHAPTER 5

THE RITE RULE #3—RAYS

Beneficial Unseen Energies Prevent Disease

Ronald, a 43-year-old dentist, came to me for a consultation as to why he was getting sick about every two months with either a cold or upper respiratory infection. He claimed that this 60-day recurring syndrome started about two years ago. At that time his practice was growing at a very high rate, requiring him to work an average of more than 50 hours per week.

After reviewing Ronald's lifestyle and recent blood tests it was apparent that his immune system was in need of bolstering. During the initial interview, I noted that he was spending far too much time indoors. He literally spent every day at the office with patients during the week and on Saturday and did paperwork at the office every Sunday.

I counseled Ronald on the value of following the 7 Rite Rules of wellness, energy, and longevity, which in his case included a tailored eating program and a regimen of natural supplements to improve his immune response. But, the most significant recommendation was for him to get outside and expose himself to the sun's pranic rays for at least an hour per day. After raising an eyebrow Ronald's first response was "pranic what?"

These are the energy rays that emanate from the sun, air, and earth. In the Orient they're called "Qigong," and in India they are called "pranic" energy rays. No matter what you call them, they play a major role in the prevention of all diseases.

I told him that even if the sun was not shining he would benefit from breathing in the air and assimilating the pranic rays that would energize his spleen and thereby bolster his immune system.

Although a bit skeptical, Ronald started right away on my program of pranic breathing and exposure, and after following the recommendations for nine months, Ronald reported that he hadn't experienced a cold or respiratory problem for at least six months. He was convinced that regular exposure to the outside air and sun's rays played a major role in overcoming his sickness syndrome. Ronald is now breathing and living The Rite Way.

The Rite Rays Rule is represented by the second "R" in the D-R-R-I-T-E S acronym. The Rite Rays Rule is the most unique of the 7 Rite Rules for wellness, energy, and longevity. In many books on health and longevity you will find some attention given to diet, rest, water, exercise, positive attitude, and the like. But most don't acknowledge the significance of invisible rays of energy known to prevent illnesses. These invisible pranic rays are also known to help overcome various forms of acute and chronic disorders.

What are pranic rays? Many types of energy rays bombard human beings on a constant basis, some beneficial and some harmful. The rays known to be of benefit are described as *pranic energies*, and are the focus of this chapter. The major sources of pranic energy emanate from the sun, air, and ground, and these rays we know have a major impact on supporting the immune system. We also know the rays from the sun promote the production of vitamin D, which is actually a hormone and has proven to be vital in the prevention of many diseases.

The Rite Rays and Pranic Energy Healing

Pranic energy can be used for healing or it can exist as a stand-alone energy emanating from the sun, earth, air, and humans. Pranic energy healing has been practiced for thousands of years in India and China. In China the practice is termed Qigong (pronounced chi-gong). In India the practice is called pranic healing (pronounced prah-nik). Pranic energy is the term used in The Rite Rays Rule because it is the term most often used in the West.

Most people are very skeptical when first introduced to these energies because they are invisible. The entire subject becomes even more mysterious when I tell people there are pranic healers who can transmit these energies through their hands. Although the pranic energies are invisible, they are nevertheless measurable with scientific equipment in the form of infrared, magnetic, and acoustical means.

The pranic energy emissions from trained holistic physicians are primarily applied to people who are in need of healing some form of chronic illness or disorder. The pranic energy rays that emanate from the sun, air, and earth are primarily recommended in order to prevent or cure chronic illnesses, although they too can be helpful in curing acute disorders.

The Sun's Energy Is a Double-Edged Sword

Everyone is aware that the sun's rays can cause damage to the skin. Damage from prolonged overexposure can be as simple as a sunburn or as serious as skin cancer. However, in my experience, skin damage is more prevalent with those who are shown to have high amounts of internal toxicities that come to the surface of the skin during overexposure. If sufficient damage is incurred, repeated exposure eventually promotes a skin cancerous state. The sun is like anything else beneficial; there is always potential for creating an adverse condition with overexposure. Anyone can overdose on any number of other good things like water, oxygen, and even exercise. However, these beneficial substances, consumed in proper amounts, are not only helpful, but they are absolutely essential. This is clearly the case with pranic energy emanating from the sun.

The classic adage by Socrates "everything in moderation nothing to excess" seems appropriate regarding sunlight. Solar pranic energy, in moderate amounts, has proven to invigorate the entire body and promote optimum wellness. You can absorb the sun's pranic rays in two different ways: sunbathing with exposure to sunlight for about 30 to 60 minutes depending on the latitude and time of day, or drinking water that has been exposed to direct sunlight for several hours. However, in order to produce sufficient amounts of vitamin D, direct exposure to the skin must occur. For the most beneficial effect and to produce the most vitamin D, expose as much skin as possible—the more the better. For most other benefits, getting outside for at least a half hour per day is effective. If you live in an area where sunbathing isn't practical year round, drink water throughout the day that has been exposed to the sun for several hours. If you live in an area where getting outside in the sun isn't practical due to the weather, then you can take supplements with vitamin D3, 2000 IU daily. If you can't get outside for at least a solid half hour per day, you can gain the exposure in increments if it's more convenient.

Outside Air Has Potent Ions from Pranic Energy

Illness prevention is a core value of The Rite Rays Rule and a major benefit of regular exposure to pranic energies. Solar pranic energies help convert outside atoms to negative ions (atoms with an extra electron) and are beneficial and not generally found indoors. Indoor air often contains atoms lacking electrons and therefore is a source of disordered energies contributing to breathing problems. Also, inside air from duct work systems found in forced air heating and air conditioning systems are often loaded with dust, dust mites, mold, and other microbes, all of which may explain why Americans incur more than five colds or respiratory infections annually.

In order to obtain these beneficial ions and energy rays one must limit the amount of time spent in airtight homes, office buildings, and vehicles. Beneficial ions and pranic energy is all around us and contained in outside air. Even though the sun may not be shining, people can still get sufficient pranic energies by getting outside for at least a half hour each day. Keeping a window open in the bedroom can also help serve to supply beneficial ions from air prana during the evenings.

Your Bioplasmic Body Helps Absorb Air Prana

Air prana is absorbed by the lungs through breathing, and is also absorbed directly by the energy centers of the bioplasmic body. The bioplasmic body, often referred to as the etheric body, is that invisible luminous energy that surrounds and interpenetrates the physical body and extends beyond it by four or five inches. People who are clairvoyant are known to have the capability of actually seeing this etheric body in the form of an aura. The energy centers of this etheric body are called *chakras,* which are spinning vortices that surround each of the endocrine glands.

The pranic energy from the outside air and the solar pranic rays are literally absorbed by the etheric body and transmitted to the various chakras surrounding the physical endocrine glands. The absorption of pranic energy by the endocrine glands and the spleen helps the body prevent many chronic diseases from occurring.

Earth Prana Also Plays a Health Role

Another form of pranic energy, called "ground prana," is also contained in the earth. It is actually energy from the sun that has been absorbed by the earth and transformed slightly to give it a violet hue. This energy can be absorbed through the soles of the feet and occurs automatically without any conscious effort. Walking barefoot on grass or bare ground will substantially increase the amount of ground prana absorbed by the body.

One can learn to consciously draw in more of all three sources of pranic energy: ground prana, air prana, and solar prana. With this energy absorption process you can expect to experience increased vitality, capacity to do more work, increased immune response, and resistance to disease.

Humans Can Manipulate Pranic Energy

Pranic energy can be projected from one person to another for healing purposes. It can also be moved and channeled in the body with a system called acupuncture. At the heart of this system lies the science and practice called Pranic Energy Healing. It has been scientifically proven that energy emitted from the hands of certified pranic healers has cured many types of chronic illnesses including cancer, asthma, arthritis, dementia, and other disorders. These healers typically spend several years in training learning to focus and use this energy to heal chronic disorders.

Up until recently, Qigong and or pranic energy healers were primarily only found practicing in the East, but within the past few years several Eastern Masters have taught many Westerners, including myself, how to generate and manipulate pranic energy. The vast majority of Western doctors have never heard of pranic energy healing and many have expressed serious doubts concerning its validity when exposed to the concepts of invisible energies and etheric bodies.

However, I can assure you, from personal clinical experience and controlled laboratory testing, that pranic energy healing works for some acute and many chronic conditions. It is very likely that the general population will be hearing more about this marvelous healing process in the near future.

"Faith sees the invisible, believes the unbelievable and receives the impossible."

—Corrie Ten Boom

I admit, when I was first introduced to the concept of pranic energy healing, I was somewhat skeptical. I never had a full conviction about its healing claims during all my research over a seven-year period. However, once I was actually trained on how to generate magnetic cleansing and radiant healing pranic energies, I became a believer. My belief in the power was completely solidified when I actually felt these energies in the palms of my hands and demonstrated an ability to remedy many different types of disorders.

Claims of Unseen Energy Rays Breed Skepticism

When electricity was first brought to the public's attention, there was a great deal of skepticism and doubt as to its existence. The doubt was due primarily to the inability to see this mysterious power. In a similar vein, people who described radio and television rays carrying sound and pictures were described as crazy—until the public saw that it was possible.

As Master Choa Kok Sui relates in his book, *Miracles of Pranic Healing*, there are people who are clairvoyant, and with the use of their psychic facilities, have observed that every person is surrounded and interpenetrated by a luminous energy aura called the bioplasmic body. He posits, just like the visible physical body, it has a head, two eyes, two arms, and looks like the visible physical body. Clairvoyants call it the etheric double, or etheric body.

He further states that the word "bioplasmic" comes from *bio*, which means life, and *plasma*, which is the fourth state of matter; the first three being solid, liquid, and gas. Plasma is ionized gas, or gas with positive and negative charged particles. He makes a point of not confusing this with blood plasma in that bioplasmic body means a living energy body made up of invisible subtle matter or etheric matter. In fact, some even suggest that to avoid confusion the term "energy body" should be used to replace "bioplasmic body." (The terms *energy body*, *bioplasmic body*, and *etheric body* can be used interchangeably.)

Science Proves Existence of Prana

It is interesting to note that science, with the use of Kirlian photography, has proven to the general public that the energy body can actually be seen and verified. With the aid of Kirlian photography, scientists have been able to study, observe, and take pictures of small energy body entities, like the energy body radiating from the fingers.

Kirlian photography, developed by a Russian scientist, actually exposes a human hand directly to special film. Upon development a person can see the energy body clearly radiating from the physical finger. It is through this energy body that pranic energy is absorbed and distributed throughout the whole physical body.

Prevention of Ill Health via Pranic Energy

One of the best and proven ways to prevent illnesses is to bolster the immune system through transmitting pranic energy to the spleen. The additional energy will help prevent or overcome common colds and the flu. To accomplish this energy boost, simply expose your back to the sun for 15 to 30 minutes a day. It is the middle of the back, the eighth thoracic vertebrae, which has a direct nerve connection to the spleen. This can be done clothed or unclothed; however, you can adjust your exposure to be longer or shorter depending on the amount of clothing you wear. It is the energy body, which surrounds the physical body, that facilitates the absorption of the pranic energy from the sun and thereby transmits its flow to the spleen. The energized spleen will now produce the needed white blood cells to support the fight against invading virus, bacteria, and other pathogenic entities which are known to cause many illnesses.

Tibetan Master Djwhal Khul promotes several additional benefits of bolstering the spleen. In his book *Esoteric Healing*, he claims the body's focus for the distribution of energy for its very life is the spleen. In the spleen, the negative life energy of matter and the living energy of the positive etheric energy body are brought together. This process is facilitated by promoting the absorption of pranic energy from the earth. Lying directly on the ground with bare skin, or walking on the earth with bare feet, or sitting in a mud bath can supply great pranic energy absorption value and result in significant therapeutic results. This pranic therapy from the earth is likened to a life stream that energizes and holds in coherency the integrated physical body. In cold climates where it might not be practical to expose bare feet to the earth, you can still gain the same benefits by getting outside for as long as possible. Go jogging, walking, ice skating, skiing, or sledding. Most importantly, get out of your house, office building, or car for as long as possible. You won't get direct earth prana, but you will gain energy from the sun and air.

According to Djwhal Khul, the stream of pranic energy vitalizes the individual atoms and cells of the physical human body and supplies an obvious uplift in electric energy.

Gaining Perspective on Radical Concepts

This entire discussion of pranic energy may seem radical and really too strange to believe. However, as the boundaries of holistic medicine and traditional Western medicine collide, several Masters have predicted that the subject will be taught in most medical schools in the twenty-first century. They also believe the Soul and the etheric body will become a subject of formalized study in many universities in the future. There is every reason to believe that science will be able to prove and substantiate with further accepted methods the idea that the Soul and the etheric body do, in fact, exist.

The concept of an etheric body extends far beyond an energy aura surrounding human beings. According the Masters of ancient wisdom, it actually surrounds and interpenetrates every atom, molecule, mineral, plant, animal, planet, solar system, and galaxy in the universe.

In the discussion of applied kinesiology in Chapter 1, Dr. Hawkins postulates that the reason testing for truth with kinesiology works is due to the interconnectedness of everything in the universe. In other words, when a muscle goes weak in response to the untrue answer to a question it can be rationalized that the individual's etheric body is connected to the universal energy. The universe ultimately knows the truth and tells the body. The body responds by going weak when the answer is false.

Djwhal Khul, in his book *Esoteric Psychology,* published in 1934, predicted that near the start of the twenty-first century a method will be developed to prove the existence of the Soul. He also posits that an increasing number of people will actually be able to see the etheric body (aura) that is in fact a part of the Soul's energy manifesting a discernable and vivid special coloring.

Although not dealt with in this chapter on The Rite Rays, Djwhal Khul has written several treatises on seven energy rays that permeate the universe, and he predicts they will eventually be studied by all psychologists in order to understand the unique rays associated with the each human Soul, personality, and physical body.

The Sun's Rays Have Other Positive Health Effects

Recent studies have shown that many diseases such as multiple sclerosis, osteoporosis, and depression can be directly linked to insufficient amounts of vitamin D. Scores of studies have proven the association of direct sunlight correlates with the production of internal vitamin D, which is now known to act as a powerful hormone. This hormone is responsible for helping to metabolize calcium into bones, protein into proper myelin covering of nerves, and for promoting proper amounts of neurotransmitters in the brain to help prevent depression.

The Rite Rays Are Vital for Human Existence

We now know the sun has been given a bad rap over recent years. Those people whose bodies are filled with toxins have problems being in the sun, and those who are generally free of toxins thrive on its emitted rays. Additionally, research studies have shown that people who live in northern latitudes with less sun exposure have more incidents of depression, osteoporosis, and other serious illnesses. Seek the sun. If you live in a less sunny area of the country or world, getting outside as often as possible will help combat these statistics. Supplemental vitamin D3 will help as well.

In many respects The Rite Rays Rule could be considered as crucial for optimum health, in that it should now be accepted that the physical body cannot maintain high levels of energy and wellness without the exposure and absorption of these energetic rays. They are essential if one is seriously aiming to reach physical immortality.

CHAPTER 6

THE RITE RULE #4—IMBIBEMENT (H_2O)

Water: The Best Drink

With her pallid skin, dark bluish smudges under her eyes, and stooped posture, Iris looked years older than 36, and with the constant fatigue and headaches that were plaguing her lately, Iris felt older, too.

"At first I thought it might be the stress of my job," she said, casting her pale gray eyes down to the hands clasped in her lap. "I'm a pediatric nurse, and it's not always easy to stay detached. In fact, a couple of the kids just about broke my heart. But the other nurses in my unit say the job's no worse now than it was when I started ten years ago. They're the ones who told me to see you. I wasn't going to, until my husband said I'm so busy taking care of sick children that I don't bother to take care of myself."

I reviewed Iris's medical tests and questioned her extensively about what she ate and drank, among other lifestyle factors. Her tests indicated a pathogenic yeast condition, which was one of the causes of her fatigue. The other main cause, based on bio-impedance results, was dehydration: Iris drank maybe one glass of water a day. I told her it didn't matter how many times she went to the soda machine; her body needed pure water in order to be properly hydrated.

I put Iris on a cleansing program to kill the yeast, a new food plan to supply the protein she lacked in her diet, and most important, a regimen of drinking much more water. In addition, she was to eliminate or reduce other beverages like sodas and coffee. When she came back to see me after two months, Iris had reclaimed her health, and it showed. Brimming with newfound energy, free of headaches, her skin glowing, and the dark circles under her eyes gone for good. Iris learned how good she could look and feel by living The Rite Way.

The Rite Imbibement Rule is represented by the letter "I" in the D-R-R-I-T-E-S acronym. Violating this rule can be a major cause of many chronic illnesses.

The principle emphasizes the importance of drinking the right amount of good water. The essence of the Imbibement Rule is captured in the phrase "the solution to body pollution is through proper dilution." Proper dilution requires about $^1/_2$ ounce of water per pound of weight. I recommend drinking in small sips often enough throughout the day to equal $^1/_2$ ounce per pound of body weight. For example, if you weigh 150 pounds, you need 75 ounces of water. It also means that other liquid intake, such as coffee, alcohol, or carbonated soda, requires an additional equal amount of water to dilute the pollution created. On the positive side, fruits and vegetables should be factored in as helping to properly hydrate, and generally 70 percent of their total weight per day can be added to satisfy the $^1/_2$ ounce water per body pound rule. For example, 70 percent of 2 pounds of fruits and vegetables equals approximately 25 ounces of water.

Imbibing the Rite Amount

Imbibing simply means taking in liquids, and in this chapter I emphasize that water is the Rite liquid of choice (proper amounts of oils are described in Chapter 3). As simple as the principle of drinking water may seem, I see patients violate it. The lack of proper volume can contribute to a wide range of serious chronic illnesses, as shown in the illness prevention matrix in the Introduction. When we look at all the illnesses the 7 Rite Rules can prevent, there's a clear major relationship of improper imbibement to all chronic illnesses.

Need more evidence on the relative importance of water and its impact on bodily health? Consider this: a human being can only exist for three days without water, whereas the body can live for forty days without food.

Many health books mention water, but most don't give sufficient emphasis to the vital importance of drinking the proper quantity of water on a daily basis. The most popular recommendation of drinking eight (8 oz.) glasses of water a day is in many cases simply not enough. Many people erroneously believe as long as they are not feeling thirsty the body is properly hydrated. When you feel thirsty, your body is already dehydrated. You should not let it get to this stage.

In order to help relate to this rule of imbibement, let me give you an example of what I do on a daily basis. My weight of 180 pounds requires 90 ounces of water a day. I front-load the amount of water in the morning in order to facilitate proper bowel movement by pouring 16 ounces of reverse osmosis water into a blender, adding two bananas weighing ¼ pound each. I sip this mixture, with a protein powder, over a 15-minute period while listening to relaxing music. Then, I typically eat half a grapefruit with a weight of 4 ounces, followed by 1 cup of sprouted grains covered with 6 ounces of berries and 6 ounces of soy milk. While exercising for 1 hour, I drink another 16 ounces and for lunch, I have 16 ounces of a vegetable salad. With a total of 65 ounces through lunch my challenge is to timely imbibe another 25 ounces (at 8 ounces a glass, that's a little more than three glasses) during the balance of the day. When you learn to love water, this amount presents no problem. On most days I will consume at least two or more fruits after lunch and a 20-oz bottle of water will fulfill my daily requirements of 90 ounces.

Total water needed: 180 pounds x 1/2 ounce = 90 ounces

Total water consumed:

16 ounces of water in the a.m.	16
Soy milk = 6 ounces with breakfast	6
8 ounces of bananas, 4 ounces of grapefruit, 6 ounces berries=18 ounces from fruits @ 70% water=	14
16 ounces of water during exercise	16
16 ounces of a vegetable salad @ 70% water =	13
2 whole ¼ pound fruits @ 70% water =	6
20 ounces of water after lunch	20
Total ounces:	91

Americans are generally drinking plenty of juices, coffee, sodas, wine, beer, and liquor. However, in order to achieve the Rite level of imbibement for proper health and longevity, it is essential to be drinking sufficient amounts of water to keep the body properly hydrated. To maintain proper hydration, a minimum of 1/2 ounce of pure water for every pound of body weight must be imbibed daily. The water contained within foods such as fruits and vegetables can also be included in the total daily input.

Is there Such a Thing as Too Much?

From time to time you may see an article about an athlete who drank so much water that it produced a toxic effect. Is this something you need to worry about? No. Pulmonary edema can occur when the respiratory system is suffocating from a lack of air due to drinking too much water. Although possible, this condition is rare among average people. There have been cases where competing bikers or other extreme sports competitors, who were taking salt pills, overdosed on water while in the midst of competition. However, it's extremely rare and not something to worry about as long as you stick to the formulas I provided above.

Quality Matters

The quality of water is also important. Ideally water should be placed through a reverse osmosis process in order to properly purify it and not remove the essential trace minerals. For example, the liquid found in fruits and vegetables is water that has been pulled up through the roots into the body of the plant in a process called osmosis. In this process the water is actually purified of all entities except for the nutritious trace minerals. It is a wonderful process that removes all toxins as it passes up through the various membranes in its journey to the heart of the fruits and vegetables. In the act of filtering out impurities, the membranes let the micro-nutrients such as trace minerals pass. Fortunately, technology has been able to virtually duplicate this process mechanically with synthetic membranes and make the pure water output available to the general public. Whenever possible, reverse osmosis water should be selected because it is preferable to all other forms of liquids.

The easiest way to get reverse osmosis water is to install a water purification system in your home. Most manufacturers make reverse osmosis systems in a wide range of sizes and prices. See your local telephone or Internet directory to find someone near you who can install a system. To find bottled water made with a reverse osmosis process, simply look for a notation on the label regarding reverse osmosis.

Why Reverse Osmosis Water Is Best

It is a fair question to ask what is wrong with tap water, bottled water, or distilled water. Taking the last one first, drinking distilled water is fine on a short-term basis. For example, if you're on a body cleansing program, distilled water will help facilitate the process of removing toxins in that it will act as a virtual vacuum cleaner as it moves through the body. This is because distilled water has no minerals, not even trace minerals, to impede its cleansing action. However, this cleansing action, used over sustained periods, can cause an electrolytic imbalance in the system. Distilled water will remove the essential trace minerals that the body needs for proper functioning of the intestines, liver, brain, and other organs that depend on proper electrolytic conditions. I would recommend you not consume distilled water on a regular basis for more than 7 days.

Bottled Water May Not Be Suitable

Many people believe that drinking bottled water is probably better than tap water, and in some geographical areas this may be true depending on the toxins and additives your municipality supplies. With most bottled waters, however, there could also be toxic concerns unless it has been purified by reverse osmosis. Tap water in many communities should also be held suspect for many inherent pathogens and chemical additives such as chlorine and fluoride. Generally, bottled water and tap water are not recommended for those who are sincerely interested in optimizing their health and maximizing their longevity. When buying bottled water, just make sure it clearly says on the label that it's produced through a reverse osmosis process. (Dasani is a popular brand, for example.) Additionally, make sure the number "1" is on the bottom of the bottle. This ensures the plastic is inert and stable under a wide variety of conditions.

Well water, if it is free of adverse bacteria, can be as good as reverse osmosis water, but many wells today are not measuring up to minimum sanitation standards. Well water should be tested for heavy metals and adverse microbes by a reliable laboratory on at least an annual basis. (Giardia Lamblia is a common parasite found in contaminated water and helocobactor pylori bacteria is also frequently found in well water. Both of these pathogens can cause serious health problems.) And one final note, if you re-use water bottles (to fill with your own reverse osmosis water perhaps for a workout) make sure you clean them thoroughly with lemon juice, grapefruit seed extract, or another anti-microbial solution between uses. Repetitive sipping will tend to build up an accumulation of bacteria and therefore the bottles should be cleaned before being refilled.

Why Is the Volume of Water So Important?

Drinking sufficient water is necessary to maintain bodily functions. Proper hydration is so critical for health maintenance that the body employs a dominant crisis water management system. Most people and many doctors are not aware that this critical body management system exists. According to Dr. Batmanghelidj in his book *Your Body's Many Cries for Water*, the crisis water management system ensures that a strict rationing of water reserves is maintained until the body receives unmistakable signals such as lack of thirst and timely imbibement that it has gained access to an adequate water supply. This crisis management system is a complex multi-level water rationing and distribution process that monitors every function of the body to ensure proper water flow. This system provides the only way of making sure that proper amounts of water, and its transported nutrients, first reach the more vital organs.

The Brain Has Priority for Water

Dr. Batmanghelidj emphasizes that one of the significant processes in the body rationing phase is the complete severity with which some functions are monitored so that one structure does not receive more than its predetermined share of water. This is true for all organs of the body. Within these systems of water rationing, the brain function takes absolute priority over all other systems. The brain, for example, will send out unmistakable thirst symptom signals, sometimes in the form of headaches, when tolerances are nearing limits.

Unfortunately, most people do not realize the stress factors created within the body's water management system when water is under-consumed. In our society, as stated earlier, many think that tea, coffee, juices, and sodas are okay substitutes for the purely natural water needs of the daily stressed body.

Drinking Just Any Liquid Is Not the Answer

It is true that coffee, tea, sodas, and sports drinks contain water, but they also contain solutes that act as dehydrating agents. The process of dehydration means that the solutes not only deplete the water they are dissolved in, but also take more water from the reserves of the body.

Triggering of a dehydration condition is critically linked to the formation of many chronic health problems. Dr. Batmanghelidj shares this view and believes that medical doctors are not taught about the many critical chemical roles that water plays in the body. (Although a cynical view, Dr. Batmanghelidj believes this is so because most medical schools are overly influenced by the pharmaceutical companies that have little interest in preventing chronic health problems.) For whatever the reasons, the general public is also obviously not realizing this critical water connection. Other signals of inadequate water supply may involve severe backaches due to a lack of hydration in the cartilage between each vertebrae, leading to an increased risk of pinched nerves. Constipation is also a condition signaling that there is probably a lack of proper hydration.

The Public Is Hooked On Problem Beverages

Today the general public craves and is dependent on all sorts of beverages that are commercially manufactured. Children would rather have soda and juice and can become dependent on the sugar and caffeine. They take these habits with them as they mature. It's not uncommon to see many adults hooked on various coffees, teas, and carbonated or caffeinated sodas. Others are hooked on alcoholic beverages like beer and wine. These poor habits turn into self-imposed restrictions on the body's water management system.

Why Isn't Water Consumption Promoted Vigorously?

It is interesting to speculate as to why the vital importance of proper water volume has not been given its needed emphasis in the health media. Generally speaking, other than the water bottling companies, no commercial interests benefit from promoting the proper volumes of water. As a matter of fact, there are a great many more forces, as stated above, working against the whole notion of proper water volume imbibement. The consumption of bottled water is on the increase primarily because of concerns about the impurities contained in tap water, but little attention is given to the bodily volume needs of water.

Moreover, the increased consumption of sports drinks also misses the point of satisfying the body's need for adequate levels of pure water. Sports drinks contain solutes that actually contribute to dehydration, because more water is required to remove the solutes. The bottom line here regarding exercise and sporting activities is that the body actually needs added reverse osmosis water in order to compensate for loss incurred during perspiration.

A good rule to follow is to weigh yourself before and after exercising. If you lose weight over the course of your workout, you should be drinking more during exercise or be sure to compensate for the loss by following the ½ ounce per pound rule.

More Reasons for Getting Hooked on Water

To make sure this water issue is well anchored in the reader's mind, it's worthwhile to mention that there are dozens of research findings that show dehydration eventually leads to serious loss of bodily functions. Dr. Batmanghelidj believes this can mean that various sophisticated signals given by the body during severe and lasting dehydration are often translated as symptoms of disease with unknown causes. He claims, and my clinical experience supports his claim, that misidentifying hydration-related issues is one of the most basic mistakes of traditional Western clinical medicine. It has prevented medical practitioners from making a proper diagnosis of conditions and causes, and thus they are unable to advise proper preventive measures or offer simple physiologic cures for some major diseases in their patients.

The Grape versus the Raisin Analogy

As stated in the case study at the start of this chapter, a bio-impedance device can accurately measure the hydration level at the cellular level. Knowing how much water is contained within the cells versus extra cellular water is important. An excellent way to help visualize this condition is to view a healthy cell as a plump grape and one that is unhealthy as a dried-up raisin. The cause of the dried-up raisin cell is due primarily to an excess of toxin solutes outside the cell, acting through osmosis pressure, causing the less dense liquid inside the cell to flow through the cell membrane to the denser outside liquid. Some of the very best ways to help ensure proper cellular hydration is to avoid toxins, drink reverse osmosis water, and eat plenty of fruits and vegetables that contain trace minerals. Following this practice will help achieve and maintain proper penetration and inter-cellular hydration.

Cellular Hydration Is a Major Bio-Marker of Aging

More than 80 percent of my practice is devoted to wellness and longevity concerns with my patients. The longevity aspect is often referred to as anti-aging. A major bio-marker (one among several dozen other bio-markers) is called the phase angle. A phase angle is a measurement of how much liquid is contained within the cell; the higher the number, the healthier the cell. This higher number generally correlates with a younger biological age. For example, a 65-year-old male with a phase angle of 5 or 6 would generally have a biological age comparable to his calendar age of 65. However, a 65-year-old male with a phase angle of 8 or above could place him at a biological age in the early 40s (depending on the measure of his other bio-markers, but the phase angle is generally considered to be one of the most important).

The measurement for phase angles is achieved with the aforementioned bio-impedance analysis device and is considered to be extremely accurate, and can be depended upon for making reliable assessments of one's biological age. Proper hydration practiced in the long term can directly affect longevity.

Many Illnesses Are Actually Due to Dehydration

When the body starts to show distress from lack of hydration or other symptoms for chronic conditions (like obesity, headaches, backaches, or constipation), it needs sufficient water for its rationing systems to distribute. However, medical practitioners have been taught to silence the signal symptoms with chemical products in the form of pharmaceuticals. Dr. Batmanghelidj believes that the various signals produced by the body water distributors are indicators of thirst or drought in particular regions of the body. If dealt with properly at the onset, with an adequate intake of water, many symptoms can be reversed and many diseases can be prevented. However, when pharmaceuticals or other commercial chemicals are used to deal with developing symptoms, complications of dehydration become unavoidable and in some cases—over a long term—the results can be fatal. At the very least, they can drastically shorten the body's lifespan.

Dr. Batmanghelidj claims that the importance of proper hydration should actually be viewed as a shift in thinking by today's health care system. It is incredibly important to alert doctors and patients to the recently understood signs of dehydration in the human body. This major difference in mindset will require doctors to change their thinking about the solid matter (solutes) protein, carbs, and fats as the most important regulator agents of bodily functions. Dr. Batmanghelidj can now demonstrate that the water (solvent) is far more important in controlling all functions of the body, including the activity of all solids that are dissolved in it. Up until recently, most research into the human body assumed that the water content of the body was to act only as a solvent, a space filler, and a means of transporting nutrients. However, studies have shown that every function of the body is monitored and pegged to the efficient flow of water. Proper water distribution is the only way of making sure an adequate amount of water reaches the more vital organs and that its transported elements (hormones, chemical messengers, and nutrients) do so also.

An Example of Body Wisdom in Action

The hydration process is an excellent example of innate body wisdom in action. When there is no interference from ingested solutes like refined sugars, sodas, coffee, or alcohol, the body's innate intelligence knows how to perfectly manage water intake for priority distribution. In this chapter, I've tried to present a clear case for why you shouldn't impede or block the innate management system by the use of medications or other toxins.

It has been clearly demonstrated, with many studies during the past ten years, that water shortages in different areas of the body will manifest various symptoms. These symptoms are often labeled as diseases such as asthma, allergies, high blood pressure, obesity, high cholesterol, stress depression, headaches, backaches, constipation, arthritis, dementia, and others.

As a practicing holistic doctor, one physical symptom that I look for in every patient is a darkness under the eyes. The darkness can take the form of bags or dark circles. This condition can be a major indicator of possible dehydration, and in many cases once proper volumes of water are imbibed the symptoms most often disappear.

Paying attention to these simple but crucial water imbibement relationships will benefit every reader, leading them to a life of optimum wellness, energy, and longevity and preparing them for the prospects of immortality.

CHAPTER 7

THE RITE RULE #5—
TOXIN-FREE LIVING

Toxins: The Cause of Major Diseases

I first met Tom when he was a top executive with a New York firm where I established a corporate wellness program. Several years later, Tom looked me up in California, where he was now CEO of a major high-tech company. He remembered how I had helped the CEO of the New York company and his family overcome health problems I'd diagnosed as caused by toxins. Now Tom needed the same kind of help for his own family, and I agreed to see what I could do.

Interestingly, Tom's wife Tricia, a medical doctor, was at a loss as to why she and Tom and their three teenaged daughters were suffering from chronic diarrhea, constipation, abdominal pain, and exhaustion. In addition, all of them were overweight to some extent, two of the girls had mild acne problems, and Tricia had severe arthritic pain in her hands and shoulders.

As part of my evaluation, I secured permission to check out their kitchen cupboards and refrigerator. "What dark secrets do you think you might find in there?" joked Tricia as I headed into the kitchen with my clipboard.

"Well, I suspect you may be harboring the biggest obstacles to health and longevity," I said, "namely man-made foods and drinks like cakes, pies, cookies, candy, ice cream, refined breads and pastas, crackers, chips, soda, coffee, and alcohol."

"You're kidding," Tricia said.

"I wish I were. Because after you give up all that stuff, even if you don't live longer, it may seem like it!" I jokingly replied.

Tricia chuckled. "I think we may have to make a few changes."

I had to agree. The cupboards were overflowing with packages of supermarket cupcakes, cheese puffs, chips, cookies, candy bars, and refined breads. There were at least a half-dozen boxes of sugar-laden cereals, all of which contained hydrogenated, transfatty acid oils. The fridge yielded several half-gallons of ice cream and tubs of puddings. The pantry had enough cases of sodas, beer, wine, chips, and pastas to toxify an army. As for the medicine cabinets, they were stuffed with a formidable array of over-the-counter painkillers, cough syrups, and prescription drugs.

It was challenging to convince Tom's entire family, especially the girls, that they were literally poisoning their bodies with the foods and drugs they consumed on a daily basis, but eventually they swore off their favorite poisons and embraced a new way of living. After several months, all major symptoms disappeared, and after another six months, the excess weight came off as well.

The key to success was their desire to change and their conscious acceptance and willingness to understand that refined breads and sugary snacks can be toxic in the same way as more common poisons. It was a major challenge for the entire family to recognize they were literally poisoning their bodies daily with toxins contained in the man-made products stored in the kitchen, pantry, and medicine chests. But ultimately, they learned overcome and prevent illnesses by avoiding processed products. They are now living The Rite Way.

Toxin-free Living is the fifth rule of wellness, energy, and longevity and is represented by the letter "T" in the D-R R-I-T-E-S acronym. Eliminating toxins from your body is a major component in the prevention of many chronic illnesses. Unfortunately, unless you have a strong wellness mindset, it's hard to really buy into this theory on toxins because it tends to spoil enjoyment of many products. However, I encourage all readers to spend the few minutes it will take to read this chapter. The knowledge it provides will pay off greatly in reducing the risk of many and varied illnesses. (And once you know what's lurking in those kitchen cabinets of yours, it will spoil your enjoyment of nearly all packaged products. Anyway, at the very least, it will make you much more conscious of some of the poisons you're putting in your body each day.)

Toxins, Wellness, and Longevity

When I first developed and presented my wellness, energy, and longevity rules to my patients, I discussed most toxic issues under the headings of eating and drinking principles. Others, I included with discussions of medical drugs, chemicals, environmental factors, pets, sex, and negative emotions as vehicles for the transmission of toxins. However, many of my wellness-minded patients asked for more information on the specifics of toxins and the problems they cause. It seemed the more serious my patients became about pursuing healthy lifestyles, the more interested in toxins they became. While often they would ask me for my opinion on research others would find tedious or too detailed, I began to realize that I should refocus some of my own writings to help those with a high interest get the truth regarding toxins. Some of this chapter may have more detail than you require, but it's necessary to help weed through an avalanche of misleading information on this subject. An elderly couple gave me the idea for using the D-R R-I-T-E-S acronym to incorporate all rules and help readers remember the principles. It also gave me a chance to give a separate treatment to toxins under the letter "T."

You should note one difference in the Toxin Rule. The other six rules presented in this book emphasize the positive aspects of what should be done to promote wellness, energy, and longevity, such as drinking enough water and exercising. The Rite Toxin-free Living Rule places the emphasis on what *not* to do, namely avoiding known toxins. Knowing what not to do is important in that we should all be aware of entities that can harm the body as impediments to the wonderful operation of our built-in bodily wisdom. Even if you followed the other six rules but omitted the Toxin-free Living Rule, you could seriously compromise your long-term wellness and longevity by introducing harmful chemicals, parasites, and toxic products into your body that cause chronic disease. Following the Toxin-free Living Rule will help your chances of achieving physical immortality, beating the clock in the race with medical science.

What Are Toxins?

Toxins are defined as any of a group of poisonous, usually unstable compounds comprised of "disordered molecular energy" generated by minerals, microorganisms, plants, or animals. The term "poisonous" can mean any substance having an inherent property that tends to destroy life or impair the body's wisdom to maintain health. The effect of toxins takes on a unique perspective with the term "disordered molecular energy." Disordered molecular energy exists at the molecular levels when electrons are lost, creating free radical atoms. As you'll recall from Chapter 3, these free radical atoms then steal electrons from what were previously orderly atoms. Added to this broad definition of toxins are the chemicals produced by the body and brain as a result of human emotional forces that are known to cause disordered molecular energy, leading to impediments in the body's innate wisdom. These effects can be very similar to those caused by unstable compounds and microorganisms.

As posited earlier, innate body wisdom plays the dominant role in maintaining health, that is, learning what your body needs and how to listen and respond to it. However, when this divine and powerful body wisdom is impeded by toxic disordered energy, its internal environment is primed for the establishment and growth of chronic disease. This is why I believe it is important to understand what these toxins are and how they impede the body's wisdom.

Toxins Need More Attention

When given proper attention, the Toxin-free Living Rule will literally help prevent many diseases from ravaging the human body. All disease is related to energy as it passes through the body in either excess or deficiency, and toxins by definition are in fact "disordered energy" causing energy imbalances throughout the body. And in today's environment, toxic exposure is all around us. In the United States alone, there are more than 10,000 food and chemical additives allowed into the food supply. The average American eats about 15 pounds of additives per year. In addition to colorings, preservatives, flavorings, emulsifiers, humectants, antimicrobials, and growth hormones, we consume on average over 156 pounds of sugar, over 56 pounds of hydrogenated oils, over 200 pounds of toxic meat and dairy products annually. Most may not view sugar as a toxin, but as will be shown, it is one of the most insidious and most hazardous of all substances.

Environmental toxins, secondhand smoke, alcohol, prescription and pleasure drugs, chemical by-products of industry, hidden chemicals, parasites in our food, parasites transmitted by our pets, caffeine, junk food, soda, and stress are all part of most of our lives. Each one of these entities should be viewed as suspect energies that create disorganized energy once in the body. This disordered energy results in great stress and degeneration to the organs and the immune system and will likely culminate in some form of chronic disease.

Why Risk Compromising Our Miraculous Immune Systems?

After much study and research on the immune system, we still do not fully understand how it works. However, what is known leaves most who have studied this magnificent system in awe. Instead of talking about T cells, B Cells, macrophages, and phagocytes, it can be viewed as an intricate and complex array of armies, navies, air forces, national guard reserves, swat teams, policemen, firemen, and neighborhood watch patrols. They are all working and communicating together in a cascading and coordinated effort to protect the body from entities that may harm it.

Pay Attention to What You Put in Your Mouth

Sally was sitting outside on the veranda of my clinic in California waiting for her appointment to see me. As I was walking into the clinic she was sipping on a soda and began to cough violently as she also munched on a bag of potato chips. I asked if I could be of any help and she said "Oh no, I have a cold and I get these coughing spells often. I think it's due to the polluted air here in California."

I picked up the soda bottle and the empty bag of potato chips and said "Possibly the California air is contributing to your problem, but you may want to think about the sugar and hydrogenated oils in these products as probable causes of impairing your immune system to the point where your body's ability to ward off bacteria and viruses has been seriously compromised."

During her consultation, she told me she consumed six bottles of soda daily and I said, "If you want to correct your history of chronic colds, you need to start paying more attention to the toxins you're putting in your body through your mouth!"

The National Institute of Health reports that nearly half the population is suffering from some sort of chronic health disease, and of equal significance is the finding that the average American contracts more than five colds or respiratory infections annually.

Lowered immunity is implicated in these illnesses and is also a prime factor in diseases such as arthritis, asthma, allergies, cancer, cardiovascular disease, fibromyalgia, lupus, and intestinal disorders stemming from pathogens that are in fact toxins. The emphasis on toxins may seem somewhat bewildering and overwhelming, but it is encouraging to note that the most significant negative effects can be controlled and minimized if we learn to pay attention to the products we are putting directly into our bodies through our mouths. Whether or not you eat or drink the toxic items discussed in this chapter can only be controlled by you.

While other forms of toxins such as secondhand smoke and air pollution are important and can enter the body through the skin or lungs, you may not be able to control it (unless you need to quit smoking). I'm not going to spend a lot of time talking about the uncontrollable toxins. But you do need to give your body the best chance you can, and the best way to achieve the longevity you're looking for is to stop willfully eating and drinking products that respected health practitioners and researchers know to be toxic—even though the general public may not realize it yet. And while you're worried about oral intake, don't forget that there are other groups of toxins you do have control over—those created by contact with pets, sexual connections, and negative emotions.

Become a Label Reader

As you begin to focus on the toxins you can control—and those you put in your mouth—you're going to need to educate yourself on the complex world of commercial and processed food packaging. Corporate America doesn't want you to know how bad most foods are for you and they don't make it easy for you to understand what you're putting in your body. They certainly don't label toxins on the box. What they do promote, though, are an endless number of "all natural," "fat-free," "sugar-free," "low-carb," and even "organic" packaged foods that in reality are toxic hazards.

I will try to give you as many clues as possible in this chapter to help you navigate some labels, but the best overall advice I can offer is to avoid packaged processed foods (that is, everything in a box, bag, jar, or can should be scrutinized for refined sugars and grains, hydrogenated oils, preservatives, and the like). Don't be taken in by packaging that touts products as "natural" and believe they'll be any better or safer for you to eat. Many contain more toxic refined products than their "unnatural" counterparts. Commercial "healthy" snacks are often the worst culprits with some granolas, snack mixes, and "healthy" cereals containing more refined sugar than you'd imagine.

Additionally, in terms of what is considered "organic," consumers should look for certified organic stores or products certified organic by USDA Organic, as decided by the National Organic Standards Board, or a reputable third party such Quality Assurance International.

Sugar Is a Toxin and a Major Health Hazard

This chapter covers a large number of toxins, and it begins with one of the simplest but most heavily consumed products in America: sugar.

Jimmy, a six-year-old with freckles, sat next to his mother during a consultation in my clinic. He was eating a candy bar and making strange noises, and he continuously fidgeted in his chair. He could not sit still throughout the half-hour consult with his mother. She knew I was aware of his behavior and said "He's been diagnosed as having attention deficit disorder and my other doctor recommends that he be placed on medications." I asked if she thought it was possible to wean him off all products containing refined sugars over the next several weeks. She said it would be difficult but she would give it try. Well try she did, and it paid off. When Jimmy returned with his mother three weeks later he was snacking on a stalk of celery and his mild-mannered behavior, due to the absence of sugar, was like night and day from the previous visit.

It is interesting to ask: How can a simple molecule like sugar be such a villain in the health process? The glucose molecule is only a combination of six carbon atoms, twelve hydrogen atoms, and six oxygen atoms represented chemically as C6H12O6. It is the simplest of all simple carbohydrates. Virtually everyone likes the sweet taste of sugar. In its natural state, most usually as part of sugar cane, it has plenty of hydration and nutritious fiber. When the fiber and water are stripped out in the refinement process it results in a dehydrated crystal of refined sugar. It is in fact much more accurate to refer to this crystal as a *carbo-dehydrate* rather than a simple carbohydrate. In either case, it is credited by most researchers and most respected health practitioners as a major dietary cause of many chronic diseases.

The glucose molecule differs from fructose in that a fibrous compound is contained in fructose that makes it less threatening but still concerning, depending on the amount of fiber and hydration contained in the final product. Refined crystallized cane sugar is glucose and even if it's labeled as organic and comes from evaporated cane juice, it causes the liver to send an immediate signal to the pancreas to start secreting insulin. However, fructose and many other sugars, known as glycol-nutrients, in whole foods will have an ameliorating effect on insulin secretion and also have widespread health benefits in cellular messaging and performance.

Refined sugar has been labeled by those in the know in the health field as a terrorist, and a devil with an insidious sweet taste that beguiles and addicts the user every bit as much as some drugs. Some characterize it as having a heavenly taste in the mouth but hellish consequences to the rest of the body. It has, in many cases, more long-term physical dysfunctional effects than most recreational drugs. It is known to be the major cause of tooth decay, obesity, diabetes, and is a major contributor to immune system impairment, cardiovascular and stroke disorders, and is implicated in yeast infections, chronic fatigue, and many addictive compulsive syndromes.

How Did Sugar Become the Bad Guy?

It is interesting to look at the history of when refined white sugar first appeared on the market near the start of the twentieth century. As Udo Erasmus gives his version, in the book *Fats that Heal and Fats that Kill*, people did not want to use this pure white stuff, because they were unfamiliar with it and therefore did not trust it. An artist with an advertising department invented and drew an imaginary "bug monster." The ad showed a big picture of this bug monster and the caption read: "White sugar never contains any of these." The image they created worked and sugar consumption has increased from 5 pounds near the start of the twentieth century to more than 156 pounds per person annually in the twenty-first century.

Other Refined Products Can Also Be Toxins

The refinement of sugar and its negative effects also has a parallel with the refinement of grains. Before the industrial revolution, only rich people could afford to eat white fiber-less flour. It had to be hand sifted, which was slow and hard work. As a result, degenerative diseases, which stem from deficiencies of nutrients and fiber, afflicted mainly the wealthy kings, noblemen, and aristocrats. The poor ate whole grains. Refined people ate refined products. The common man's foods were crude, like his upbringing and manners. As Mr. Erasmus tells it, "Poor people struggled to become refined." To afford refined foods was a sign of prestige. The connection between refined foods and degenerative diseases was overlooked, and the fact that refined foods actually are nutrient deficient escaped people's attention. The consequences of this problem are discussed later in this chapter.

It wasn't until the 1970s that the connection was largely made between refined nutrient-impoverished foods and chronic diseases. Moreover, it's only been the past few years that medical science is beginning to tout that refined sugar is the major culprit in creating the widespread obesity problems in America.

Sugar Is the Major Cause of Body Fat

Although the sugar-to-fat connection began to be promoted by the medical community in the '70s, the general public still is largely unaware of the conversion of sugar in the diet to fat in the body. The processed food manufacturers and their army of PR people attempt to give the impression that it is dietary fat that causes fat to be stored in the human body. Therefore, enormous advertising and packaging campaigns stress the low fat content of nearly everything on the supermarket shelves. But it is really a diversionary technique to take attention away from the continued high percentage of sugar contained in the majority of packaged and bottled products. The fact is that the majority of the population is literally hooked on it and the processed food manufacturers know it and encourage it. They can't reduce the sugar content in most products without a noticeable drop in sales. Anyone who doubts the pervasiveness of the sugar substance in our products is invited to stroll down the aisles of any supermarket and read the label of contents on the shelf items. What you'll find is that nearly 90 percent of the products have sugar added and that many will have sugar listed as the second or third ingredient on the label, meaning it's the second or third highest-percentage ingredient. Even if the label reads organic evaporated sugar cane juice, it nevertheless means the product is the simple sugar glucose, and should be avoided.

Diseases Caused By Sugar

With more than 150 pounds of sugar consumed annually on average by each person in the U.S. (the actual number as of 2000 is 156), it's no wonder we're facing an obesity epidemic. It is reasonable to predict that about one-third are consuming more than the average amount of sugar per year and those who do are probably morbidly obese. Today's definition of morbidly obese means more than height and weight relationships as represented by a body mass index, which tells nothing about the fat level inside the body. To get a meaningful understanding of obesity, a body composition measurement by either hydrostatic or bio-impedance devices is required. (These devices are available in many health clubs and clinics. Bio-impedance measures, with a low-level current, the volumes of fat, lean tissue, and water in the body.) A measurement with either of these systems will accurately show how much fat is contained in the body. The standard for optimum fat level is 15% of total body composition for men and 20% for women. Any fat level exceeding twice the optimum places the person in an obese category. Fat levels above 45% places one in a morbidly obese category.

Obesity Is a Major Disease

Obesity should be taken seriously because it is a condition that places the individual at high risk for cardiovascular disease, diabetes, strokes, hormonal disorders, immune system impairment, and some forms of cancer. The Surgeon General of the United States announced in 2001 that nearly one-third of the U.S. population is obese and that this condition is responsible for illnesses causing as many as 300,000 deaths per year.

If you examine what takes place in the body when sugar is consumed, it will help awaken your consciousness. The idea is to move those who are adversely affected from a state of denial to a level of contemplation that should result in corrective eating patterns.

Fat Is Not Just Passive Baggage

When I met with Betty, the diabetic with the beautiful café-au-lait skin weighing over 200 pounds as described in Chapter 1, I showed her a replica of what 10 pounds of fat looks like—a fabricated 10-pound yellow rubber, sticky globule. This fat globule sits prominently in my consultation room, and with the explanation of this glob being a hormone factory contributing to mood swings and other chronic problems, she got the message that helped motivate her to lose over 60 pounds of fat in less than a year. Showing Betty a virtual real-life example of the problem proved to be much more effective than just telling her about the adverse consequences of excessive body fat.

What most people do not realize is that refined sugar is converted by the body directly into a fat called triglycerides. With each pound of sugar consumed approximately 80% is transformed by the liver into triglyceride fats. These fats are stored in the body as excess energy, and are known to absorb and store large quantities of toxins and cause a great deal of increased health risks, as stated earlier. It should be realized that fat is not passive baggage; it is a prolific factory that can pump out 25 different hormones, according to endocrinologist Dr. Roger Unger of the University of Texas and Dr. Jeffrey Bland of Health Comm Inc. in Washington state. One of the hormones produced in fat cells is estrogen, which can lead to imbalances and estrogen dominance and has been associated with premenstrual syndrome, uterine fibroid tumors, fibrocystic or painful breasts, cervical dysplasia, endometriosis, systemic lupus, and cancers of the breast, uterine, and ovaries. This excess estrogen production can occur in men as well.

More directly, the ingestion of sugar causes the pancreas to secrete the insulin hormone, and when this is overdone the body's cells become insulin resistant, resulting in type 2 diabetes and causing other problems. Metabolic syndrome X, also known as insulin resistance, affects approximately 46 percent of Americans and is characterized by high blood pressure, high cholesterol, and high blood insulin and glucose levels. People with metabolic syndrome X are at greater risk of developing heart disease, type 2 diabetes, stroke, Alzheimer's disease, and for women, fertility problems.

Tooth Decay (and Tooth Repair) Is a Major Hazard

There is an additional insidious disease resulting directly from the over-consumption of sugar and that has to do with the undeniable link to tooth decay and cavities. Some may ask, "Well what is so serious about cavities? When you get a cavity simply go to the dentist and get it filled." But the problem is that the filling contains even worse toxic substances, such as mercury and silver amalgams known to be responsible for a great many illnesses. Moreover, the process prior to filling the cavity normally requires a prescription painkiller of some sort. Some studies have shown that some of these painkillers are implicated in contributing to pre-cancerous conditions and in the formation of a number of tumors. The dental association has denied these claims of amalgam toxicity and cancer-causing agents for many years; however, most health care professionals and researchers believe that avoiding putting poisonous metals and chemicals in your body breaks the link to many chronic health disorders.

Dr. Hulda Clark claims in her book *A Cure for All Diseases* that a debate still rages over mercury amalgam fillings. No one disputes the extreme toxicity of mercury compounds and mercury vapor, but the American Dental Association feels that mercury amalgam fillings are safe because they do not vaporize or form toxic compounds to a significant degree. However, health care proponents cite scientific studies that implicate mercury amalgams and other teeth replacement procedures as disease causing. For example, cadmium is used to make the pink in dentures. Cadmium is five times as toxic as lead, and is strongly linked to high blood pressure. Dr. Clark points out that occasionally, thallium and germanium are found together in mercury amalgam tooth fillings. Thallium causes leg pain, leg weakness, and paraplegia. The effects of thallium are cumulative and its major effects are on the nervous system, skin, and cardiovascular tract. (Many health researchers claim that mercury in any form is toxic and at high concentrations causes liver and kidney damage and neurological symptoms.)

Dr. Clark emphasizes that the cancer-causing or carcinogenic action of metals has been studied for a long time, although it doesn't get the attention by regulatory agencies. She mentions her thinking was influenced considerably by a scientific book entitled *Carcinogenicity and Metal Ions*, which depicts nickel compounds as one of the most carcinogenic metals. (Nickel is used in gold crowns and children's crowns.) What are your other options? You can ask your dentist about solutions including inert porcelain compounds. But prevention is always preferred over even the best of cures.

Parents Need to Teach Children the Dangers of Sugar

Rosa, a mother of five, brought her middle boy, 15-year-old Gerardo, in to see me for a weight management and chronic fatigue consultation. Gerardo, at 5 feet 7 inches and 215 pounds, wanted to play football but claimed he was constantly fatigued and too tired to attend practices.

After gaining an understanding of his health history and lifestyle, it was clear that Gerardo's consumption of four bottles of soda, four candy bars, and at least one piece of his mother's homemade cake or pie each day were the major causes of his obesity and chronic fatigue condition. His blood sugar level was far above normal and he displayed all the symptoms of a type 2 diabetic. Gerardo had five cavities filled in his molar teeth over the past two years. As it turned out, all of Rosa's children were having problems with cavities and surprisingly she claimed that she was never made aware that their excessive consumption of sugar was the major cause of fillings, and in her personal case, crowns and several tooth replacements.

While all of this discussion on the potential hazards of dental fillings, crowns, and tooth replacements might be tedious, confusing, and in some cases contradictory to what is proffered by the American Dental Association, it should serve as an alert to the benefits of preventing tooth decay. There is little controversy that sugar and the products that contain sugar and phosphoric acid like that contained in sodas are the dominant cause of the majority of decay disorders. It should also serve as an alarm to parents and educators that they should pay more attention to dental health by informing children and guiding them away from the formation of sugar habits at a young age. There are myriad disorders beyond cavities that are of concern and connected to the sugar habit. As any adult who is hooked on sugar will testify, the addiction probably started in childhood and overcoming the habit can be every bit as challenging as ridding oneself of a serious drug habit.

Diabetes

In Gerardo's case, his probable development of type 2 diabetes was a serious matter and I counseled him and his mother on the need to eliminate refined sugars and carbo-dehydrated products across the board. Beyond the cavity concerns, I let them know it was imperative to get Gerardo's blood sugar level down to normal in order to avoid insulin resistance from developing any further. The consequences of type 2 diabetes, even in teenagers, can lead to serious health problems including obesity, heart disease, chronic fatigue, and many others.

A Sugar Picture Can Be Worth a Thousand Words

I have found it helpful, when talking to people about health, to speak in terms of pictures. The image that has proven to be most effective with regard to the negative consequences of sugar is to have them think about the effects of pouring a bag of white sugar into the gas tank of a car. If you're having trouble kicking your sugar habit, visualize the phrase "gumming up the works" and the icky, sticky conditions created within the engine parts and how this is similar to the icky, sticky fat generated within your body when you eat refined sugars. In engines, impurities create excess carbon residue. Human bodies generate excess fat and hormones. These images should give you another perspective to the toxic disordered energies created from the over-consumption of sugar.

Refined Grains Are Toxins!

Refined grains have many of the same negative consequences as refined sugars. These products, made impure with over-processing and additives, are refined starches acting like sugars. Consumed in excess, they are major culprits in making people overweight and/or obese. They adversely affect blood lipids and blood sugar levels, and foster a myriad of diseases including the morbid illnesses of cardiovascular disease, cancer, and diabetes.

Whole grains, by contrast, which make up less than 5 percent of Americans' carbohydrate consumption, contain wonderful health-enhancing bran (the outer layer) and germ (the internal embryo) and are naturally found in all whole grains. The whole grain contains a perfect ratio of essential fatty acids, protein, and carbohydrates.

However, when grains are refined to make regular white flour, the bran and germ and all their healthful nutrients, antioxidants, fatty acids, and other disease-fighting chemicals are systematically removed. The majority of the food manufacturers use these refined grains to make breads, crackers, cookies, candy bars, cereals, and chips, and in most of these products they also add sugar, hydrogenated oils, and a number of fillers, preservatives, and taste enhancers. Refined grains alone cause disordered energies and add toxins to the body, and the vast majority of processed snacks also include sugar and hydrogenated oils. The combination is a major contributor to the ill health of millions of people in America and around the world.

These refined and dehydrated grains are often referred to as simple carbohydrates, but in fact as with the sugar crystal, void of water, it is more accurate to call refined grain products "carbo-dehydrates." It is this characteristic of dehydration that runs as a thread through most processed foods and it presents a classic case of adulterating previous vital and nutritious natural foods. In the case of refined grains, the adulteration is compounded due to dust, mold, and yeast spores, collected during extensive storage, resulting in aflatoxins that can literally blind the human immune system upon entering the body. For those who desire an alternative to refined grains, one should look for sprouted grain bread products without added sugar or hydrogenated oils. These healthy grain products will probably only be found in health food markets (for example, Ezikial 4:9 is a sprouted grain bread product).

Whole grains such as the kernels of wheat, rice, oats, and barley, after soaking in water over night and adding fresh fruits as a topping, is a delicious and nutritious way to consume whole grains.

Another Visualization Picture

To help picture the negative effects of refined grains, I ask patients to visualize again "gumming up the works" with icky, sticky fat production within the body but to also create an image of putting a mask on your immune system. Think of covering the eyes of soldiers on the battlefield so they cannot identify an invading enemy. Then I ask them to realize that this masking is exactly what happens to your immune system when the aflatoxins in refined grains do their dirty masking work on your "T" cells within the body. Bottom line... you're going to have more unidentified microbes attacking you and you're going get sick more often due to a degraded immune system.

Bad Oils Are Also Major Toxins!

Many patients have come to me with bad skin they descibe as "acne." One woman in particular, 35-year-old Audrey, suffered for years with terrible blemishes on her face. She was very good-looking with good features and bone structure but she was obviously self-conscious and troubled by her skin condition.

When I reviewed her diet it was clear that she over-consumed candy bars, chocolates, pastries, and french fries. I felt these were the major cause of her skin problems. These products contain distorted energies in the form of rancid and hydrogenated oils, which often cause mischief beyond poor skin conditions. In Audrey's case three weeks of avoidance of the problem foods coupled with following my 7 Rite Rules, and a tablespoon of high-quality omega 3 oils daily, cleared up her acne condition.

Sugar and refined grains get the most attention because as toxins they are responsible, by far, for the most serious and most prevalent chronic illnesses in America. But not far behind are hydrogenated products. Hydrogenation of oils is one of the most common ways of drastically changing good natural oils into bad transfatty acid oils. Unfortunately, these hydrogenated transfatty acids are pervasive in all kinds of food products, including salad dressings, crackers, cereals, cookies, breads, potato chips, chocolate, margarine, and candy. One of the major reasons food processors hydrogenate oils is to supply additional body and texture and life span to packaged products. Transfat gives crackers that buttery crisp or crunch even after they're weeks old. It's also used to help certain soft products such as margarine and chocolate hold their shape.

If you're a label reader, you'll notice that many companies tout their products as "transfat free." Why? Transfats have gotten such a bad name in the past few years that many food manufacturers have begun to remove them from their foods. As of January 1, 2006, the U.S. government required all package labels to include how much transfat is in a product. This doesn't let you off the hook, though. As large food manufacturers phased out transfats and hydrogenated oils, they replaced them in some cases with combinations of partially hydrogenated fats and new chemical additives that are just as bad.

What Are Hydrogenation and Transfatty Acids?

No matter what your opinion of the food industry, the fact still remains that the hydrogenation process has quite a few negative effects. How does hydrogenation work? It involves manipulation of oils from a variety of sources, including nuts, seeds, and vegetables with high amounts of pressure, heat, and hydrogen gas in the presence of a metal catalyst (usually nickel, platinum, or copper) for up to eight hours. This processing converts oils to transfatty acids and other impurities. The ingestion of these transfatty acids, which behave as free radicals, cause our cells to degenerate, age, and die at an accelerated rate.

Free Radicals Behave Like Terrorists in the Body!

I have used this terrorist analogy with my patients and it has proven to be highly effective in getting them to abstain from using hydrogenated products. At the risk of sounding overly dramatic, hydrogenated products are disordered energies acting like terrorists in that they literally steal electrons from healthy tissues and cells and cause a detrimental free radical chain reaction with neighboring cells and molecules.

Here's another visualization: The free radical internal effects on the body can be visualized as causing a pyrotechnic display very similar to a bursting cell if viewed through a microscope, compared to a super nova explosion in the cosmos viewed via a telescope.

Free radicals are also generated from other treatments of oils beyond the hydrogenation process. Frying and deep-frying are two major ways to cause oils to convert to transfatty acids and cause free radicals. Moreover, when oils are exposed to light and or to air there is always the risk of rancidity and resulting free radical formation. Therefore, all oils for consumption should be purchased in dark bottles and kept refrigerated and capped after opening to prevent the above from occurring.

Why Are These Bad Fats and Oils on the Market?

As I stated in the Introduction, the food processing firms are not intentionally producing fats and oils to harm us. Rather, they are not trying to produce good health promoting foods. What they obviously have as their first goal is to produce profits, and they know the public is hooked on many of their products that are processed and altered for so-called better taste, texture, shelf life, and so on. The bottom line to the consumer should be "caveat emptor," that is, the buyer should be aware and skeptical of all processed fats and oils and adhere to the warnings discussed above in order to minimize toxic effects.

Most Processed Foods Contain Toxins

By now, you may have begun to realize that in order to keep growing and commanding a larger share of the market, processed food manufacturers believe they must continue to sweeten, artificially flavor, dye, preserve, or otherwise alter food in order to maximize their manufacturing process, grow market share, and increase profits. In other words, most manufacturers process the food to whatever extent is necessary to give it a long shelf life with an appealing taste and appearance.

By now you should also have this point clearly anchored in your mind: Processed foods are more profitable to the corporations and more dangerous to the consumer for the following reasons. With much of the food value removed and dozens of preservatives added, processed foods last practically forever. When flavors, colors, and textures are synthesized, corporations are freed from dealing with the cost and bother of higher-quality foods and real ingredients. Most importantly, the foods can be designed to appeal to consumers who think they are educated buyers without undue concern and expense over the toxic effects of their processing methods. In essence, they are relying on the public relations articles planted in magazines, newspapers, and TV stories inducing you to believe that you're buying nutritious food, when in reality you're not.

Long Shelf Life Can Mean High-Toxicity Products

Shelf life is clearly one of the industry's top priorities. According to biochemist Paul Stitt, who worked for several food processors, it is not at all unusual for the freshness codes on food packages to brag that the product inside will still be in edible condition almost a year after it arrives in the store. On the surface, Mr. Stitt claims, this may seem like quite an achievement, but on reflection it is clear that these long-lived foods are not really fresh. They have merely been doctored in one of two ways: Either they have been loaded with preservatives, more accurately poisons, that ward off the growth of microorganisms, or the nutritive content of the food has been depleted to the point where no microbes could live on it. This may seem like a great scientific accomplishment, but as Mr. Stitt points out, "The microbes are after the same things in the food that your body needs and utilizes when you eat."

Examples of More Toxins from Processed Foods

Remember, toxins are poisonous disordered energies and they impede the body's wisdom from doing what is best for it. Toxins must be avoided if one is serious about maintaining and promoting optimum wellness and increasing the prospects of a longer and vibrant life. In addition to refined sugar, refined grains, and transfats, there are a variety of other well-known chemicals and additives that you should avoid.

The following substances are found in a variety of processed foods and drinks and are considered toxins. Before purchasing and or consuming processed food and drinks, make sure you read the label to determine if any of these toxins are present:

- **Aspartame and other false sugars:** Introduced as an alternative to saccharine, aspartame is an artificial sweetener that is about 200 times sweeter than sugar, and has been linked to many chronic illnesses including high blood pressure, headaches, insomnia, mood swings, extreme dizziness, brain tumors, epilepsy, allergies, and retina deterioration. Aspartame is most often found in sugar-free processed foods and drinks, most major brands of diet soda, and under the brand names of NutraSweet and Equal. Nearly all diet soft drinks contain some form of these false sugars. A number of false sugars including Splenda regularly hit the marketplace. All of them require some form of toxic processing. The only sugar substitute, other than whole fruits, that I recommend for sweetness is a Stevia solution created from a Bazilian plant and available in most health food stores.
  Dr. H.J. Edwards (a world expert on Aspartame and a diabetic specialist) summarized many diabetic reactors and claims that he advises all patients with diabetes and hypoglycemia to avoid Aspartame products. Russell Blaylock, M.D. Neurosurgeon in his book *Excitotoxins-The Taste That Kills* says "Aspartame may trigger clinical diabetes." He also claims that excitotoxins, which can be found in such ingredients as NutraSweet, literally stimulate neurons to death, causing brain damage of varying degrees.
- **MSG:** Often MSG, a popular additive for processed foods, is a dangerous neurotoxin that can cause serious brain damage. The full name for MSG is monosodium glutamate and it is a big-time toxin that should be labeled as hazardous to health.
- **Phosphoric acid:** This substance is often contained in soft drinks and is a major contributor to leaching of calcium from the bones and hence fosters the chronic disease of osteoporosis. It is also known to cause tooth decay.

- **Artificial colors and flavors:** These terms can include a wide range of suspicious substances that in most cases have toxic effects on the body. Generally the full nutrient content in the product is low because of refinement processing, particularly prevalent in breads where brown coloring is used to give the appearance of wholeness.
- **Natural colors and flavors:** Just as potentially toxic are what many manufacturers label as "natural." All "natural" often means is that the artificially manufactured flavor has some basis in a natural element.
- **Soda drinks and commercial cereals:** These categories of products are mentioned here and singled out because most of them contain immense quantities of sugar. Most soda drinks contain at least nine teaspoons of sugar and a typical box of supermarket shelf cereal can contain even more. These products are high-volume, high-profit items for food processors. For proof of profitability and revenue, look at the space given to these products on all supermarket shelves.
- **Preservatives:** Most food additives are simply a mystery. No one knows for sure what they are doing to the body but the odds are they probably cause some type of energy distortions and disease through long-term usage. Preservatives like BHT and BHA keep foods from going stale for months, but it should be realized that their real benefit is to the manufacturers, enabling them to reduce processing, shipping, and storage costs.
- **Pesticides:** Dozens of different types of pesticides are prevalent in most processed foods, animal products, and fruits, vegetables, and grains. Some are worse than others, but all in some way detract from the immune system and the body's ability to repair and reproduce new cells without mutations. This problem should be taken seriously and is one of the major reasons why only organic produce, animal products, and processed foods should be consumed.
- **Herbicides:** There have been more than 75,000 synthetic chemicals released into the environment since World War II. Less than half have been tested for potential toxicity to adult humans. Some of their names include Glyphosate, Triazine, Cyanazine,

Agent Orange, Paraquat, and Diquat, all of which are used to kill weeds and other unwanted vegetation. The problem is that trace amounts are often found on the fruits and vegetables and packaged products produced by the processed food industry. These are all to be avoided and this is another good reason for only consuming products labeled organic.

Some Final Thoughts Regarding Processed Foods

If you are eating processed foods on a regular basis, you are probably at high risk for a multitude of chronic diseases for all of the reasons discussed above. Remember the concept of "disordered molecular energy"? It is the most important reason regarding the dangers of consuming man-made processed foods. You now should recognize that food manufacturers take what was once "ordered molecular energy" in the form of hydrated real foods like grains, seeds, fruits, and vegetables and dehydrate, cook, and add whatever it takes to make them taste good and last longer on the supermarket shelves.

All of this processing results in transforming what was once health-building, organized molecular energy into disease-creating, disorganized molecular energy. It is worth repeating that all disease is related to energy as it passes through the body in either excess or deficiency, and processed foods are major creators of energy imbalances once they enter and flow through the body.

Animal Products—and Some Animals—Carry Toxins

When James came to see me at the clinic where I practice holistic healing, he was complaining of abdominal pain, fatigue, and uncontrollable diarrhea typical of a condition called irritable bowel syndrome, or IBS. For James, going out in public or accepting an invitation to dinner wasn't worth the risk that he might have to reveal his condition. He was tired of assessing his ability to participate in social activities based on the proximity of public toilets. Only 36 years old, this sandy haired, amiable man was so depressed by his curtailed social life that he was starting to wonder if life was worth living at all. "If it weren't for Sarge—he's my yellow lab," he said as he let his head drop to his chest, "I don't know what I'd do."

When I asked James to tell me about his pet, he visibly brightened as he described how Sarge would greet him at the door every day when he came home from work. It was their little ritual. Sarge would jump and bark until James knelt down and let Sarge lick his face. Sarge was by his side every moment James was at home, and James smiled sheepishly as he admitted he spoiled the dog rotten by feeding him bits of rare steak or sushi from the table and letting him sleep in his bed.

From this little bit of information, I formed my theory about the source of James's condition. A comprehensive digestive stool analysis proved me right when it came back positive for parasites, bacteria, and a yeast condition. It seems that James's lifestyle was the culprit. How? The rare meats and raw fish he frequently ate were one source of parasites; his dog licking his mouth and nose was another.

Treating James's condition was simple. I gave him herbs to kill the parasites, a plant-based medication to kill the bacteria and yeast, and some probiotics, or "friendly bacteria," to replace what the tests revealed his body had lost. In addition, I instructed him on some crucial lifestyle changes, including the necessity of cooking all meats and fish thoroughly and of eating only organic meats that are guaranteed to contain no antibiotics (which destroy friendly bacteria in the intestines). Like most people, James had no idea how important it is to have *good* bacteria in the intestines; those little organisms are what prevent parasitic and yeast infections from taking hold in our bodies.

Another important change was that James could no longer allow Sarge to lick his mouth or nose. "And that's nothing personal against Sarge," I said, "all animals that spend time outdoors have parasites, and any of us who have contact with them should wash our hands before touching our faces or our food."

After six weeks on the program, on a follow-up visit, Jim expressed a zest for life with energy that he hadn't felt for over a year. His diarrhea and abdominal pain had completely stopped and he could hardly find the words to fully express his delight in new-found energies and feelings of well-being.

I like to begin any discussion of the potential problems with high consumption of meat or other animal products by soothing the emotional response. Don't panic! If you are a heavy consumer of meat and animal products, just keep an open mind to the clinical research and I think you'll be surprised at the amount of correlation between various diseases and heavy, non-organic meat consumption.

Preventing Parasites and Other Animal Diseases

With the media coverage of Mad Cow disease (bovine spongiform encephalopathy, or BSE), its human version, variant Creutzfeldt-Jakob Disease (vCJD), and Hoof and Mouth epidemics, meat consumption declined significantly, particularly in European countries. The relatively high incidents of these diseases (compared to previous years) during the early years of the twenty-first century have served to raise the public's awareness of some of the potential hazards of consuming animal products. The purity of the meat supply has become a major concern of governments and consumers alike. If you consume meat or fish, you need to know the risks and take steps to protect yourself. It's also your responsibility to learn what you can and not panic needlessly. The facts? Depending on what and how much you eat you probably have nothing to worry about. Heat and cooking will kill parasites in meat and fish, but not prions, the proteins that carry BSE and vCJD. Even organic meat can put you at risk, but with proper handling and by avoiding brains, spinal tissue, and animal organs, you can minimize your chances for problems.

Virtually every animal has parasites; however, with proper cooking techniques most parasites will be destroyed. With this risk in mind, no animal should be consumed in its raw or undercooked state. Popular examples of these raw conditions include sushi and sashimi and raw beef dishes like steak tartar. Consuming either places you at high risk for tape worm and other types of parasitic infections.

Animals with Added Hormones, Chemicals, and Additives Are Toxic

Most beef animals consumed today spend their last months in overcrowded stockyards, fattened on high-calorie feed loaded with medication and additives. Factory farm-raised pigs and chickens rarely leave indoor barns as they are fed, medicated, and moved for slaughter. Their flesh is tainted, chemicalized, and adulterated. Most are raised in environments surrounded with pesticides and herbicides, and nearly all are shot through with growth hormones and slow-release antibiotics. After slaughtering, the meat is often preserved with nitrates or nitrites. All of these are toxins and are passed into the human body at the dinner table.

Many people believe the government is inspecting animal products at a high level of confidence, but only one in every quarter million animals are tested for toxic chemicals. More importantly, the government doesn't consider synthetic bovine growth hormones (such as rBGH or rBST) or most medications in meat today toxic. The National Academy of Sciences reported in 1985 that federal inspection procedures are inadequate to protect the public from meat-related diseases. A similar report in 1999 indicated that the public is still significantly exposed to meat-related diseases. For example, one-third of chickens inspected have salmonella bacteria. Most federal inspectors (75%) said they simply will not eat chicken because of their experiences. Testimony from a former FDA official to a Senate investigating committee claims the risk of food poisoning from chicken is so great that package labels should contain mandatory handling and serving warnings.

The estrogen-based growth hormones fed to the animals may seem harmless to humans, but even the ingestion of trace amounts have been shown in many foreign scientific studies to have a strong connection to abnormal human growth patterns. Some foreign countries are beginning to impose restrictions on imported meat due to the heavy use of synthetic growth hormones. Many studies here in America have also implicated these estrogen-based hormones as possible culprits in causing the premature development of breasts and the start of puberty in 9- and 10-year-old girls. There are also many studies that implicate the estrogen-based hormones with a connection to higher rates of breast cancer in women.

The feeding of antibiotics to virtually all animals, including poultry, is another practice that seems reasonable in that it may help protect the animals from bacterial infections. However, when these antibiotics are ingested by humans, even in trace amounts, they act as toxins killing the good bacteria that reside in the intestinal system. These good bacteria protect us from the pathogenic growth of adverse bacteria, yeast, and some forms of parasites. Now the consumers of these animal products are exposed to higher risks of intestinal diseases such as irritable bowel syndrome, Crohns disease, and other imbalances associated with overgrowth of pathogens.

Dairy Products Are Not Free of Pathogens

Dairy products contain all of the toxins mentioned above, and contrary to popular belief, are not even the most desirable source of calcium. Absorption of calcium from most dairy products is poor due to pasteurizing and high fat content, and the unbalanced relationship of phosphoric acid acts as a toxin, in that it promotes the leaching of calcium from the bones. It turns out that the very best way to get calcium absorbed into the body is almost exactly the way cows do... eat green grass or green leafy vegetables.

Dairy products also can contain parasites ranging from protozoa to a vast array of adverse bacterial conditions. Bacterial infections are considered to be parasitic in that they live in and feed off the human body and can create enormous damage to various bodily systems. According to Hulda Clark, in her book *The Cure for All Diseases*, all milk should be boiled before consumption to protect against Salmonella and Shigella bacteria. She also recommends avoiding yogurt and cheese, which cannot be boiled. These may seem like extreme measures, but if your immune system is not at optimum levels even small amounts of adverse bacteria can cause severe pathogenic reactions. Studies have shown this reaction in children who drink cow's milk and subsequently show patterns of ear infections and respiratory disorders. What are your alternatives? I recommend soy and rice milks over cow's milk if you consume dairy products. Eggs should be organic. If there are any concerns about a compromised immune system, you should avoid dairy products completely.

Commercially Slaughtered Animals Have More Toxins

Another type of toxin in animals comes from the "fight or flight" response. When animals enter the slaughtering pens or slaughterhouse in a state of fear, hormones and uric acid literally flood their bodies. For example, when an animal isn't processed quickly enough in a meat processing plant, it can sense the presence of death through odors and sounds, causing a state of shear terror. This condition causes the adrenal hormones and uric acid to saturate their flesh.

Although the adrenal hormones and uric acid may not be viewed as toxins, their effects may cause aggressive behavior, fear, and a lack of sensitivity in humans.

All Animal Products Should Be Organic

Animal products can be good sources of protein and if you're going to consume them, you'll want to avoid the condition of added toxins by man. Serious consideration should be given to purchasing only those products that are labeled USDA Organic or that are certified organic by a third party such as Quality Assurance International. With these assurances, you can be reasonably confident that the animals in question are fully vegetarian fed and that ranchers and farmers have not added any antibiotics, growth hormones, or other additives. You can also be fairly certain the animals have not been exposed to pesticides or herbicides. Organic products typically cost an additional 15 to 20 percent, and good organic meat can be even more expensive, but over the long run the reduced risks of ill health will justify the added expense.

Pet Parasite Warnings

I want to touch on one more area of toxin exposure from animals. As I mentioned in the earlier story about James and with IBS, we discovered that some of his problem had to do with his beloved lab, Sarge. Quite a few parasites are transmitted by animal contact, in particular pets like cats and dogs. Many of my patients with parasitic infections have pets, and when I ask if they let the animal lick their hands and face they often answer "yes." Letting your pet's saliva come in contact with your nose or mouth seriously raises the risk of parasitic infection. The risks go higher when pets spend any time outdoors.

The simple act of petting an outdoor animal raises an additional risk. You should wash your hands thoroughly with soap or an anti-microbial wipe before you touch any food or bodily orifices.

All of these toxic issues take on added importance if you have any kind of compromised immune system. The toxic conditions I discuss in this chapter are all potential immune system detractors and probable impediments to the wonderful and divine body wisdom.

Drugs, Alcohol, and Caffeine Can Be Toxic

Dark-eyed Maria, attractive but slightly overweight, was a successful attorney, dedicated to serving the Latino community in Los Angeles. She was referred to me after years of re-occurring yeast infections. She was also recently diagnosed with fibromyalgia.

Maria was nearly in a state of tears, with a look of agony, as she described her current condition of pain that radiated over her body. Her pain was particularly acute in her thighs, arms, and shoulders to the extent where her husband Carlos couldn't even touch or embrace her without causing rejection of some sort. He was beginning to wonder what was going on.

Her medical doctor claimed that fibromyalgia was an auto-immune disease with no known cure and he prescribed several pain relief drugs to help ameliorate the symptoms. However, she claimed the drugs were making her feel nauseated and came to me for another opinion. Maria was also on a drug called Flagyl to help her deal with a two-year re-occurring yeast infection.

The consultation uncovered the fact that Maria was on and off Flagyl for several years and that it was over this period that symptoms of fibromyalgia also started to appear. Having dealt effectively with many yeast infections and fibromyalgia cases, I related to Maria that the cause of her disease was likely due to a condition referred to as "leaky gut syndrome." This could mean that fecal material is leaking into the bloodstream, causing the immune system to build antibodies to the protein in the fecal material and subsequently attacking similar protein found in the myelin coverings over nerves. Her nerves were in effect comparable to electrical wires with frayed insulation and accounted for the intense pain whenever she was touched.

After reviewing a comprehensive stool test, my theory was confirmed that Maria indeed had some serious yeast and bacterial imbalances in her intestinal system. Correction of the yeast condition was accomplished with probiotics, taken to restore good bacteria, and the ingestion, for six more months, of special natural products repaired the mucosal lining of her intestines, correcting the "leaky gut syndrome." As her fibromyalgia disappeared, her husband Carlos came in personally to shake my hand for helping Maria overcome her pain and allowing them to resume a normal life.

Medical Drugs Can Be a Double-Edged Sword

Prescription drugs have been essential in saving lives and have helped shorten the duration of many acute diseases. However, extensive research shows that virtually all medical drugs, even when correctly prescribed and consumed, will have toxic disordered energy side effects and probably, ultimately, shorten your life span. In most cases, commercial drugs only suppress symptoms and do not really cure the cause of a chronic illness. If you are currently taking prescription medication for long-term control of a medical problem, as an alternative you should seek out a doctor who will pursue the cause of the chronic illness and treat it with natural substances like whole foods and natural supplements and offer advice for lifestyle changes to prevent a re-occurrence.

In Maria's case, her medical doctor had prescribed an antibiotic for treatment of her yeast infections. While this treatment may reduce or eliminate a pathogenic level of yeast, it will in all likelihood also kill the friendly bacterial flora residing in the intestinal system, creating an environment where adverse bacteria and parasites can grow unimpeded. In Maria's case, I felt it also led to development of further illnesses such as her leaky gut syndrome. This condition has been implicated as a likely cause of arthritis, lupus, and fibromyalgia.

Prescription medications, especially taken incorrectly or in combination with other medications, can cause a myriad of problems, even death. At issue is the fact that we just don't know how they react in the body short term with many other medications and substances, or how they react in the body long term. Allergic reactions, side effects, and combination reactions can cause you to end up sicker than you were before you tried to treat the original illness. Additionally, the AMA cites that a minimum of 100,000 deaths a year are caused by prescription drugs, giving additional weight to the argument that prescription drugs aren't always the optimum solution many in the pharmaceutical industry would have you believe.

Recreational Drugs Are Never the Answer

Whatever the reason for using recreational drugs such as alcohol, marijuana, cocaine, speed, opium, or any number of others, you can be sure you are causing toxic disordered energy to impede your body's wisdom. The drugs are most likely causing some major side effects that will lead to ill health and a shortened life span, whether you recognize them or not. These sorts of drugs offer false hope and short-term remedies for anxiety, relaxation, or stimulation. They don't help you forget your problems, find self-confidence, or reduce depression. Anyone who is addicted really knows this in their heart, but most often is in a state of denial. Professional help is almost always needed to help people overcome a drug habit. While there are long lists of reasons to stop recreational drug use, taking care of your body by ridding it of toxins and disordered molecular energy are some of the most important.

Alcohol Destroys Cells and Promotes Body Fat

Richard, at 360 pounds on a 6 foot 2 inch frame, was treated for morbid obesity and a drinking problem during a 12-month period and lost over 60 pounds under my lifestyle coaching program. Richard had a friendly and engaging personality and I spent many hours counseling him on The Rite

Way to overcome his excess weight and drinking. However, in addition to these issues, Richard had a severe back problem and his medical doctors deemed it could now be helped by surgery after his substantial weight loss. The operation was not as successful as the doctors hoped and Richard, an alcoholic who hadn't had a drink in over a year, started to indulge again. He quickly ballooned back up to over 360 pounds and a blood test showed that his liver was on the verge of collapse. He was also showing signs of memory loss and severe fatigue. Richard was literally destroying his body and mind. Although I was able to convince him to enroll in a 12-step program through Alcoholics Anonymous, Richard died three months later from cirrhosis of the liver.

Alcohol is a drug and, although it is legal and sometimes touted as having beneficial coronary effects, it is a toxin and killer of cells. It impedes the body's wisdom in a major way by unleashing free radicals on the liver, intestines, immune system, and brain. It also causes lasting chronic illnesses that will likely shorten life spans and lead to painful deaths. Even if you drink in moderation and think you're safe, you need to understand alcohol also is converted to sugar and eventually to fat by the liver and is therefore open to all of the diseases mentioned earlier regarding simple sugar carbohydrate consumption. Diabetes, cirrhosis, dementia, obesity, yeast, wrinkles, and cellulite are all conditions known to be connected with alcohol usage.

Support groups that help people deal with alcoholism claim that those who consume more than one drink a day are candidates for being classified as alcoholics. They often factor in any number of other profiles including family history, body weight, and gender. Whether or not you are at risk of becoming an "alcoholic," you need to understand the very real risks involved to your body. Additionally, addiction has serious implications for mental, emotional, and physical degeneration. If you are addicted to alcohol or believe you might be at risk, seek professional help to recover.

Caffeine Is an Irritant and Destroyer of Nutrients

Like many of mankind's pleasures, there is good and bad news about caffeine. In Sandy's case we have a bad news story with a happy ending. Here is an attractive woman, 30 years old, with a successful career as a vocalist and entertainer. However, Sandy was extremely worried about having constant irritability in her throat and problems with acid reflux in her esophagus and stomach. Sandy was concerned that her career as an entertainer might be over. She also noted regular bouts of migraine headaches and feelings of jumpiness and occasional heart palpitations. Her consultation revealed that she consumed three to four cups of coffee daily. I asked Sandy if she had ever tried to abstain from coffee and she claimed every time she tried her headaches became intolerably severe. I suggested that she try again with gradual reduction over a 10-day period and that she could expect to have headaches for about three days after completely abstaining from coffee. When she came back to see me four weeks later, she reported nearly all of her symptoms had vanished, including her major concerns of throat and stomach irritability.

Some of the health problems associated with caffeine are well established and include migraine headaches, irritability, stomach and digestive disorders, anxieties, and hypertension. Coffee drinkers hate to hear this, but caffeine is an addictive stimulant, and as such it should be considered as a drug that can cause the body to become over-stimulated. This over-stimulation can lead to sleep disorders, digestive disorders, nervous disorders, and heart problems indicated by increased palpitations. In excessive amounts caffeine can produce oxalic acid in the body, leading to a wide range of conditions waiting to become chronic diseases. It can act as a toxin in the liver, restricting and disrupting its function of wrapping and disposing of other toxins. It can also constrict arterial blood flow. It leaches B and C vitamins from the body and contributes to increased stress effects as a result. Excessive use contributes to depletion of essential minerals, including calcium and potassium, and affects the endocrine glands, causing hormonal imbalances that have been implicated as a major factor in the growth of breast and uterine fibroids in women, and prostate disorders in men.

To wean yourself off of coffee, see my advice above, keeping in mind that caffeine is insidious and can be found in more than just coffee, tea, and soda. To flush it out of your system, drink equal amounts of water to compensate.

More Challenges to the Body's Wisdom

Knowing that alcohol is a depressant, and caffeine is a stimulant, imagine for a moment what it might be like if you had to play the role of your body's wisdom trying to keep all systems functioning properly and in balance with continued use of either of these substances. Ask yourself if these substances are likely to have an adverse effect on energy balancing and the functioning of your body's wisdom. Most of my patients, who are suffering the ill effects of either one of these toxins, will show some resistance to eliminating them from their diet. However, when I ask them to imagine how their body's wisdom is going to deal with the known adverse effects of these substances, I quite often get good compliance after reflecting on the difficulties of dealing with the challenges listed above.

Toxins Resulting from Negative Emotions

One of the last toxins to cover is one produced inside the body. A serious amount of toxicity can be generated from negative emotions. Whether you are affected by stress, anger, frustration, or anxiety, this is an area that is difficult to measure and therefore does not get the needed attention from the present-day medical community. However, I believe it's a major cause of chronic illness. Fortunately, more doctors are now recognizing that emotional disorders often lie at the root of many chronic illnesses. What is the cause? Negative emotions can represent or manifest as a blockage in the solar plexus energy pathways and can result in a wide range of gastrointestinal and headache disorders. It's significantly better for your body to address these issues through education and lifestyle changes, preventing serious illness in the long run.

One useful technique to eliminate toxins caused by negative emotions is to work with a doctor trained in the science and art of pranic or QiGong energy healing. Properly trained healers are able to scan the etheric energy body with their hands and detect where a congestion may exist in the physical body. The congestion can often be cleared up with appropriate use of magnetic energy from the energized hands of a certified energy healer. After the diseased area is detoxified or decontaminated, a trained healer can then radiate the appropriate energy to the affected area and restore or reenergize the pathways.

In some respects this methodology has a number of energy manipulation similarities to the well-known therapy of acupuncture that has been used in China for millennia.

Anger Can Evoke Destructive Storms in the Body

Monica came to see me for my opinion on what could be in her diet that might be causing her stomach pain and indigestion symptoms. As I was reviewing information about her eating habits and lifestyle, she received a cell phone call from her teenage daughter who apparently had done something she shouldn't have. Monica, who was well-dressed and neat and appeared to be very rational with a pleasing personality, went into a frenzy, carrying on for several minutes with a high-pitched screaming tone while her free hand and head flailed in quick animated movements. After hanging up she apologized for the interruption and said that her daughter was driving her nuts. I asked how her stomach was feeling at this moment and she claimed it felt like it was being torn apart.

I asked Monica to rethink her opinion that something in her diet was causing her stomach pain and to consider employing some of my emotional self-management exercises. Monica agreed to follow my exercises and after six months she had learned to prevent most of the emotional outbursts that had plagued her in the past, and as a result she also noted a complete absence of stomach pain.

Looking at the problem from a comparative standpoint, let me note that anger and other negative emotions can generate dysfunctional energy imbalances every bit as damaging as toxins ingested orally. I believe it is useful to view emotional responses as having a liquid characteristic that influences the emotional body to vibrate at destructive levels. The vibrant emotional action can take the form of liquid acid reactions in the stomach and/or the intestines and can have other far-reaching effects on the liver, pancreas, heart, and brain. Why do I refer to it as a "liquid response"? It's an esoteric concept: all emotional reactions are related to the emotional body and are characterized by its liquid properties as opposed to physical body solidness, mental body gaseousness, and etheric body ionized plasma.

In some respects, a severe emotional reaction can be compared to a large hurricane or cyclone sweeping through parts of the body. To help my patients understand the effects of this destruction on cellular and organ structures, I ask them to visualize tornado forces and the resulting damage and destruction to buildings and life on the surface of the planet. Out of the 60 trillion cells in the human body, every anguished expression can easily result in thousands of disruptions and deaths to cellular structures. This may seem like a small percentage in view of trillions of bodily cells, but when you factor in the damage it causes and the time and energy it takes the body to repair this damage, you can see the effect of ongoing negative emotional reactions and the havoc and destruction they can wreak over time.

Severe Stress Can Have Toxic Effects

Doctors often point to the stress factor as the culprit for causing many modern-day diseases. There is abundant medical research to show that the brain, under conditions of negative emotions—hate, fear, panic, rage, anger, depression, frustration, and so on—can produce powerful changes in the body's chemistry. Dr. Walter Cannon, in his book *Bodily Changes in Pain, Hunger, Fear, and Rage*, describes how the body produces toxic poisons when under siege of negative emotions. Researchers have produced overwhelming evidence that prolonged anger, depression, and grief can have negative energy effects on the immune system, reducing the body's ability to combat hostile microorganisms or to cope with abnormal changes in cell growth.

It is clear, in view of many research findings, that we have the ability to make ourselves ill. But now, on the positive side, there is credible research accumulating that we can also make ourselves well. Chapter 9 discusses your internal health and the research supporting the value of a positive attitude. However, some of these findings are really not new. Hippocrates, thousands of years ago, insisted that his students give full weight to the emotions both as a contributing cause of disease and as a factor in recovery.

More recently in a book entitled *Esoteric Healing*, Master Djwhal Khul claims that at present many humans are astrally polarized and that the emotional sentient nature is all-powerful in the masses. From the emotional state of consciousness much concerning individual ill health can be deduced. He further states as a basic generalization that personal physical trouble has its seat in the emotional body, and that this vehicle of expression is a predominant predisposing agent in the ill health of the vast unthinking public. The dynamics of this dominating factor take the form of a stream of desire energy that can lead to wrong emotional attitudes and a general unhealthy condition of the astral body. This is an important factor in producing discomfort and disease according to Djwhal Khul. He further claims this is due to the fact that the vital etheric and physical bodies of the masses of humanity are governed primarily and swept into activity through the action of the astral (emotional) body.

Agitation in the astral body through any violent activity under stress of temper, intense worry, or prolonged irritation will pour a stream of astral energy into and through the solar plexus center, and will galvanize that center into a condition of intense disturbance. This next affects the stomach, the pancreas, the gall duct, and bladder.

Violent Criticism and Dislikes Should Be Avoided

The tendency for some to criticize others, to violent dislikes, and to hatreds based on a superiority complex, produces much of the acidity from which many people suffer. Stomach ills are closely tied up with the desire aspect of the physical body. These ills find expression in the eating and drinking of that which is desired, leading subsequently to those attacks of excess bile secretion and liver disorders to which so many are prone.

Much more could be said regarding the toxic effects of negative emotions, but I believe the major points have been made which clearly indicate that regular conscientious efforts should be pursued to gain control of one's emotions. Of course this is easier said than done, and Chapter 2, "The Rite Way to Change for Life," deals with this issue in a fair amount of detail.

Transmitted Toxins via Human Contact

When Patricia came to see me she had been divorced for about eight months and was suffering from strange conditions that she had never experienced before. They included blisters appearing around and in her mouth and blemishes that showed up on her torso and legs. Patricia had auburn hair and sparkling green eyes, was very neat and good-looking, but was surprisingly shy and slightly introverted. Her health history revealed that she had joined a dating club and that she had been going out with several different men at least once or twice a week for the past several months.

After reviewing her blood, saliva, and urine tests it was clear that she was harboring several types of bacteria, viruses, and yeast entities. Although Patricia claimed she was not having sexual relations with any of her dates, she said that she was frequently involved in heavy petting sessions. I also discovered she was extremely stressed and experiencing bouts of depression after the divorce, which made her less resistant to transmitted microbial entities.

After clearing up her problems, my prevention advice included developing an intimate emotional and mental relationship with awareness of each man's health history before getting involved in intimate physical contact. Although this approach seems very clinical, it is much better to have this knowledge before intimate contact than have to spend time and money, with associated health risks, at a clinic for treatment of microbial diseases.

It's important to realize that a wide range of toxins can be transmitted by sexual contact. In this case, Patricia was suffering from skin lesions due to these foreign bacteria, viruses, and yeasts. While standard sexually transmitted diseases (STDs) such as syphilis, gonorrhea, and herpes cause significant medical problems, I want to introduce you to a broader concept involving personal cleanliness. I'm not advocating a compulsive level of cleanliness, but want to give more attention to the potential adverse consequences of many and varied intimate human contacts. You may also be at risk in some forms of plain casual contact. If you are involved with one partner on a regular basis, your body will build up immunities to what were at first foreign microbes.

Every human being carries unique forms of bacteria, virus, molds, and possibly some type of animal parasites. Some have immune systems that can tolerate and successfully fight off exposure to new forms of invaders of various species. However, when many new microbial forms are encountered on a frequent time-compressed basis, complications can often arise. With frequent and heavy exposures to microbes, the immune system can be overwhelmed, allowing pathogens to take hold. Whereas given more time between exposures, the immune system would have the ability to recognize and build immunity to the new pathogens. These types of microbes can be transmitted through sex and various sexual contacts including mouth to genital, hand to genital, and mouth to mouth contacts. With mouth to mouth issues, the reader should know that the typical oral cavity houses more types of microbes than the vagina or intestines, with more than 600 species of bacteria. Added to this might be parasitic, viral, and yeast entities. Therefore, those with less than optimum immune systems are at high risk for contracting some type of infection stemming from adverse microbial entities. And of course the risk goes up with more varied and increased intimate human contacts.

Toxin-Free Living Leads to Longer Life

All of these toxic issues take on added importance when there is a compromised immune system involved. The toxins presented in this chapter are detractors to all systems and in particular the immune system, and overall are probable impediments to the proper functioning of the wonderful and divine bodily wisdom.

It should be clear at this point that a toxin-free life plays a major role in preventing all diseases. Giving this rule its deserved attention will pay large dividends in promoting wellness, energy, and longevity with increased prospects for achieving immortality.

How to Be Tested for Toxins

If you have concerns that you may have toxins or parasites in your body, the appendix lists a number of ways to be tested. Depending on what substances you feel are involved there are a number of ways to be tested. The tests may require hair, stool, blood, saliva, or urine output and the appendix explains how tests can be conducted in any area of the country. If your regular doctor can't test you, then seek out a licensed holistic doctor for an examination and advice.

CHAPTER 8

THE RITE RULE #6—EXERCISE

Proper Movement to Prevent Disease

As a result of an article I wrote on how specialized endocrine exercises could prevent many diseases and help increase wellness and longevity, Edward, 49, and Elaine, 46, came to see me. Edward's mother had had a stroke 12 months ago and was recently placed in an assisted living care center. They were very dismayed after visiting many centers and seeing thousands of patients like her unable to care for themselves.

Edward and Elaine, although having some wellness issues, looked like the picture of health, resembling in some ways a happy doll image of Ken and Barbie with thick, light brown hair and radiant smiles. As I discovered later, from their many referrals, they were respected and active members of the community and were leaders in several charity and social organizations. After raising three children they wanted to enjoy the rest of their life and were intrigued with the prospect of living a long, disease-free life. They eagerly embraced and followed the 7 Rite Rules of wellness, energy, and longevity, enrolled in the endocrine exercise program, and also took the introductory exercise programs covering aerobic and anaerobic movements. Over the past five years they claim to have never been sick and never felt better. They have referred several dozen patients to The Rite Exercise Program, all of whom have learned to live The Rite Way.

"The joy of being alive and moving is a true measure of life."

—Anonymous

The sixth rule of wellness and longevity is represented by the "E" in the D-R-R-I-T-E-S acronym. The exercises in this rule cover the lung, the heart, and the muscle groups that will benefit from aerobic and resistance movements illustrated in this chapter. Additionally, I also provide several exercises critical to maintaining hormonal flow through the endocrine glands. All of these exercises are important for maintaining optimum wellness, energy and longevity.

Use It or Lose It!

At the start of the twenty-first century less than 20 percent of the American population actually exercised on a regular basis, although you wouldn't believe it from the images you see on television and in magazines. Even general observations of people jogging, riding bikes, and joining health clubs leave the impression that the majority of the country may be heavily involved in exercising. But the numbers are actually very low. When researchers ask why people don't exercise, the reasons are varied. Answers include "I don't have time," "I'm too tired," "Health clubs are expensive," "Health clubs are meat markets," "I feel uncomfortable at health clubs," "My feet hurt," "My back hurts," "I don't like to sweat," "I don't see a need to exercise," "I'm happy the way I am" and "I get plenty of exercise at work because I take the stairs instead of the elevator."

People who don't believe they need exercise tend to be in a state of denial about adverse consequences. In some respects the non-exercisers are victims of what psychologists would term "cognitive dissonance syndrome," where they will build a list of reasons for not exercising whenever they see someone else doing it. For example, if they see someone jogging their mind starts to generate all the negatives against jogging, which might include "Jogging makes my knees hurt," "I need new jogging shoes and can't afford it," "I can't jog in this cold weather," "It is nonsense to risk exposure to all those gas fumes," or "I could fall or sprain an ankle." All of these reasons can be viewed as rationalizations and cognitive dissonance enhancements that tend to support the decision for not exercising. Even worse, people who are used to this denial tend to associate with others who discount the benefits of exercise, creating more excuses for not getting active. Whether it's a spouse, friend, or partner, often even the best of intentions for change are made more difficult by our inert enablers.

Many benefits are known to emanate from various forms of exercising. Conversely, there are many known adverse consequences of inactivity or non-exercising lifestyles, and in summary it boils down to simply "use it or lose it." "Using it" can help promote your body's physical immortality and prevent any number of illnesses, as described in the Introduction.

Aerobic Exercise Offers a Myriad of Benefits

Aerobic exercise (also known as simply "aerobics") is the most popular type of exercise, generally including any type of sustained movement such as walking, jogging, cycling, or swimming. The most obvious benefit comes from raising the heart rate, perspiring, and increased breathing, which in turn causes an increase in the metabolic rate and a subsequent increase in the burning of calories. Perspiring leads to a wonderful detoxification process through the skin. Another benefit comes from the release of hormones called beta endorphins. These hormones are released from all muscle groups involved in the aerobic movements and serve to cause a subsequent increased flow of neurotransmitters in the brain. All of these actions result in a feeling of mild euphoria, a high of sorts, which tends to motivate the exerciser to want to do more exercising in the future.

Exercise Reduces Heart Attacks and Strokes

A sedentary lifestyle contributes to 250,000 deaths in the United States per year. According to the monthly *John Hopkins Medical Letter*, this is about 12 percent of the total coronary heart disease deaths per year. When combined with poor diet, physical inactivity is the second most significant underlying cause of death in America. People who do not exercise have a 30 to 50 percent greater risk of developing high blood pressure and are almost twice as likely to develop coronary heart disease (CHD) as those who are active.

Aerobic exercise can help turn around these grim statistics. A recent study in the *Archives of Internal Medicine*, for example, followed more than 30,000 people aged 20 to 93 for 14 years. It found that those who consistently exercised, played sports, or biked to work were significantly less likely than their peers to die of any cause over that time period. The highly active people were about half as likely as the inactive subjects to die during the study, and the moderately active people were about one-third less likely. This benefit increased with age, especially in women. Other studies have confirmed a similar effect in men. Research has also documented that aerobic exercise reduces the risk of CHD-related death by about 25 percent in people with established CHD.

> *"Life is like a bicycle: You don't fall off unless you stop pedaling."*
>
> —Claude Pepper

Aerobic exercise has also been linked to a reduction in strokes, the third leading cause of death in America. A report in the *Journal of the American Medical Association*, based on data from more than 72,000 women aged 40 to 65, found that performing 30 minutes of moderate to vigorous exercise, including brisk walking or jogging almost every day, cut the risk of ischemic stroke (strokes caused by narrowed or blocked blood vessels) by 30 percent. The risk of hemorrhagic stroke (caused by bleeding into or around the brain) was cut by 20 percent. Similar data are not yet available for men, but it seems reasonable to assume that results will be approximately the same.

Exercise Reduces Risks for Diabetics

Aerobic exercise reduces the risk of developing diabetes and may increase the life span of people with this condition by helping insulin work more efficiently, thus lowering abnormally high blood glucose levels. A recent study in the *New England Journal of Medicine* examined more than 500 men and women at risk for diabetes by virtue of their being middle aged, overweight, and having high blood glucose. Those who received counseling on techniques for effective weight loss, making dietary changes, and boosting exercise were 58 percent less likely to develop diabetes. Other studies show that exercise reduces complications and extends life after diabetes has developed.

Exercise Reduces Risk Related to High Blood Pressure

The blood pressure lowering effects of aerobic exercise are due to a variety of reasons. In general, regular aerobic workouts increase the amount of blood ejected from the heart with each contraction. The workouts also promote more efficient use of oxygen. Both of these effects lead to lower blood pressure during exertion and while at rest. Recent research also discovered that aerobic exercise helps prevent age-related deterioration of the endothelium (lining of the blood vessels), which can lead to atherosclerosis (fattening and hardening of the arteries) and the formation of blood clots. Exercise helps to avert this type of degeneration by ensuring that enough nitric oxide is available. This substance, which is produced by the endothelium, signals the blood vessels to relax when the heart needs more blood.

Sweating Is Glorious

One of the major goals of aerobic exercise should be to obtain a level of speed and time whereby a perspiring condition exists for a minimum of 10 minutes. Sweating should be viewed as a highly desirable condition that indicates a high level of caloric burn and also facilitates a natural cleansing and removal of toxins from the respiratory system, fat cells, and skin systems of the body. Generally it requires about 20 minutes of rapid walking or slow jogging to create a state of sweating, depending on the ambient temperature. Proper hydration during the walk or jog will help promote the sweating process. A sip or two of water every five minutes is generally sufficient to do the trick. A lack of ability to sweat generally indicates a need for more salt and/or B6 vitamins in the diet. If this does not make a difference, the addition of regular amounts (1 ounce daily) of ginger root into the diet almost always makes a noticeable difference in the ability to sweat.

I have found that perspiring for at least 10 minutes is extremely important for proper cleansing and caloric burning and reduces the reliance on measuring the heart rate to achieve the above benefits. Of course if there is any concern of heart problems, follow proper precautions and visit a doctor who is knowledgeable about the ins and outs of exercising.

Aerobic Pace Can Be Overdone

There is an important consideration regarding the wasting of lean muscle when a sustained high pace of aerobic exercise is maintained. Here there are a number of theories as to the most effective speed in relation to heart beats per minute. Some physiologists claim that subtracting your age from 220 gives the heart rate to be maintained throughout the entire aerobic workout. By this method, for example, a 50 year old should maintain a heart rate of 170 beats per minute (220 – 50 = 170). However, my research has shown that depending on one's body mass and composition, this pace at one-half hour or more can cause the burning of lean muscle. A more conservative and effective calorie burning method is to measure the resting heart rate, and go no faster than 80 percent of the resting rate added to the resting rate. Therefore, if the resting rate is 70 beats per minute, 80 percent of this is 56, and when added to the resting 70 beats the total is 126. Therefore, 126 beats per minute should be maintained throughout the 30-minute aerobic workout.

For a person with a resting rate of 70 beats per minute, the latter pace will not burn lean muscle because the glycogen has not been exhausted from the muscles. With the first method, requiring a heart rate of 170, it is highly likely that even if the glycogen levels are at maximum levels in the muscles, the glycogen will be exhausted within 30 minutes. Glycogen is produced from carbohydrates and is the clean fuel for moving the body and is stored primarily in the muscles. Once the glycogen supply is exhausted, the body will start to burn lean tissue in order to keep the muscles working. Some people believe it is desirable when more calories are burned at the 170-beats-per-minute rate because it also results in a loss of weight. However, if the body composition is measured after this workout, it will be shown that lean body tissue as a percentage of total will most often be reduced and total fat percentage will most likely have gone up. This undesirable condition occurs because the additional calories burned at the higher pace have actually come from burning lean muscle.

What Seems Like Good Exercise Can Have Bad Effects

The troubling aspect for people on a weight management program is that too much of the wrong exercise can actually hamper the ability to burn fat. They may be losing weight, but it is not healthy fat weight loss. If this condition continues with excessive muscle loss, one will be hopelessly caught up in a vicious cycle contributing substantially to a yo-yo syndrome. One will be wondering why with all the exercising and good eating programs, they are unable to reduce the fat around the abdominal section, thighs, and or the gluteus maximus area.

The key points to remember are to slow the heart rate down to the most effective level, make sure the body is kept hydrated, and to employ an anaerobic weight training program for muscle enhancement and maintenance.

Meat Eaters and Soda Drinkers Beware

Aerobic exercise should be engaged in at least three times per week, and if more is performed the benefits will continue to follow. However, another potential downside to extensive aerobics will sometimes show up in the knees, particularly to those who are meat eaters or soda drinkers. Knee joint deterioration is more apt to occur when there is an overabundance of phosphoric acid in the diet, and meat and soda are two major offenders in this regard. If joint pain is a problem, one might consider using a step machine that will reduce the stress pressures generally felt in the knees.

If joint pain is still a problem, then bike riding or swimming should be engaged as an alternative.

Foot problems are also more prevalent with joggers and this is why it is so important to be fitted with a superior pair of jogging shoes that present absolutely no impingement signs, such as pinching or abrasion. Ill-fitting shoes can cause blisters, microfractures ("shin splints"), and a wide variety of other foot, ankle, leg, hip, and back soreness.

Exercise Programs Must Be Managed with Clear Goals

One of the big challenges in the pursuit of any exercise program has to do with making the exercise a regular habit. I view myself as a coach, particularly with my overweight patients, and here my advice is to counsel them on the merits of preparing a written schedule that can be prominently posted on the refrigerator or on a desk. This exercise routine should be viewed as an important lifestyle element and given priority to ensure proper compliance. Your family members and loved ones should know your schedule and do whatever they can to encourage your compliance. Surround yourself with people who want to help you succeed, not people who want to see you fail because they, too, are sedentary. Set goals and set a schedule for your exercise. If you see yourself as a morning person who wakes up with plenty of energy, you may want to schedule a morning workout of brisk walking or jogging at least three times a week. If you have a flexible lunch hour and your place of work is near a health facility, this may be a good time for you to schedule a regular workout. The point here is that no matter what time you select, it is critical to commit yourself to this schedule and view it as a priority in maintaining a healthy lifestyle.

Anaerobic Exercise Is Required to Burn Fat

Anaerobic exercise is often called resistance training, where the object is to maintain or slightly build lean body composition. To maintain lean muscle, you should do resistance training exercises for a minimum of two 25-minute sessions per week. If the goal is to build a little lean muscle, then plan at least three to four 25-minute sessions weekly. Plus, this entire muscle maintenance or building process enables you to burn fat while sleeping. In other words, the anaerobic exercise sends the message that the affected muscles are in need of repair and the fat cells in proximity serve as the energy source to make this repair happen naturally.

Lean muscle tissue adds healthy weight to the body because lean muscle weighs more than the same volume of fat. In addition, higher volumes of muscle are able to store more glycogen and serve athletes particularly well, helping extend competitiveness because of the increased storage of fuel. (The body starts to burn lean muscle tissue once the glycogen stored in the muscle is used up.)

Another excellent reason for following a regular routine of muscle resistance exercises is to help bolster the maintenance of bone mass. Women, especially, can see severe drops in bone density after menopause, which can lead to osteoporosis as well as other problems. Osteoporosis is a growing problem in America, particularly among women, and even a mild amount of regular weight resistance could serve to prevent this disease from becoming a chronic health problem.

The specific muscle training exercises needed are very simple and easy to perform and can be done at home with very little expense. However, I have found that those who make a financial commitment to a health club membership are somewhat more likely to stay with the program. Whether working out at home or in a gym, the following routine will serve to maintain and build muscle tissue.

If you are on any medications or are experiencing any symptoms that are causing you discomfort, you should get approval from your doctor before doing this exercise or any of the other exercises depicted in this book.

Basic Fat-Burning Muscle Training Routine

Simply stated, there are 10 basic exercises that can be performed in less than 25 minutes. There are four body movements for the lower half, one for the middle, and five for the upper body. If you use a health club, a staff member can usually direct you to the appropriate equipment. If you do these exercises at home, I recommended you purchase some light weights with Velcro straps to fasten to the ankles for lower body workouts and to the wrists for upper body movements. Generally, 10 percent of your total body weight should be sufficient for each arm and 15 percent for each leg for good resistance. There is no need for grunting and straining to achieve desired muscle maintenance. In this case, more weight doesn't always do the job.

The following sections present the basic steps for a good fat-burning and muscle training exercise routine.

Gluteus Maximus

The lower body should be worked first, and squats are highly effective for firming up the rear end. The key point to remember here is to make sure that the knees do not extend past the toes when at the bottom cycle of the squat. Also, at the completion of 15 repetitions you should consume one sip of water, followed by two more sets of 15 repetitions with a sip of water between each set.

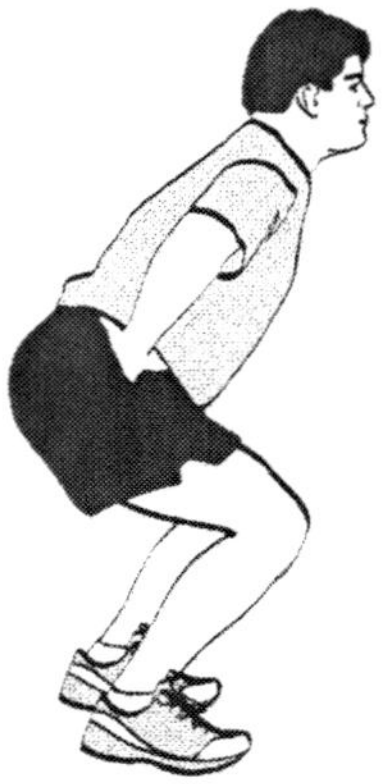

Squats
Squeeze gluts when rising.
Do three sets of 15.

Quadriceps

This group of four muscles is located at the front of each thigh. You can effectively exercise them using leg weights (or a machine) and by moving one leg up and down while in a sitting position. Begin with your heel on the floor and raise the leg from the knee until extended in a straight line, perpendicular to your torso. I recommend using 15 percent of body weight on each leg for good resistance. If you don't have access to a machine, try leg weights that attach to each ankle with Velcro or other straps.

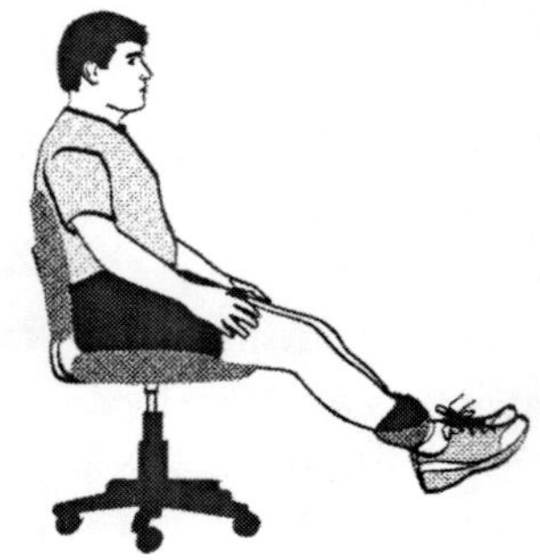

Leg Raises
Use leg weights. Do three sets of 15 on each leg.

Hamstrings

This group of muscles is located at the back of each thigh and can be effectively exercised by doing a reverse curl with each leg while standing. With both feet on the floor, extend and curl one leg as far back as possible. Repeat on the same leg 15 times, and then switch. Fifteen percent of body weight on each ankle should be sufficient.

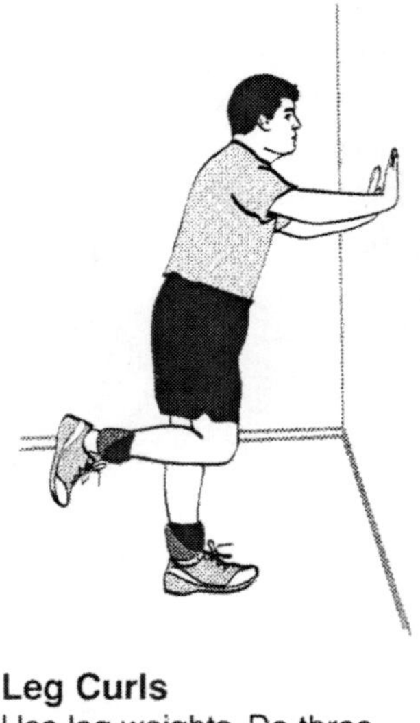

Leg Curls
Use leg weights. Do three sets of 15 on each leg.

Calves

Calves are the group of muscles located at back of the bottom of each leg and can be exercised without the use of weights by simply doing toe raises and using your body weight for resistance. For this exercise, stand erect, then simply raise your entire body on your tip toes and lower again.

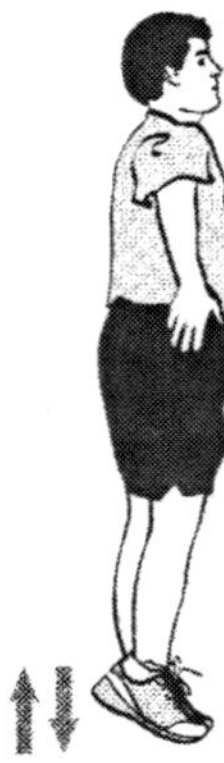

Toe Raises
Move up and down on your toes. Do three sets of 15.

Abdominals

Your abdominals are located in the front of your midsection and can be sufficiently exercised by simply performing crunches (similar to sit-ups). In a crunch, you lie down and hold your hands behind your head, then lift your head and neck about 10 inches off the floor. The abdominal muscles should tighten while you raise your head and neck. Do three sets of 15 repetitions.

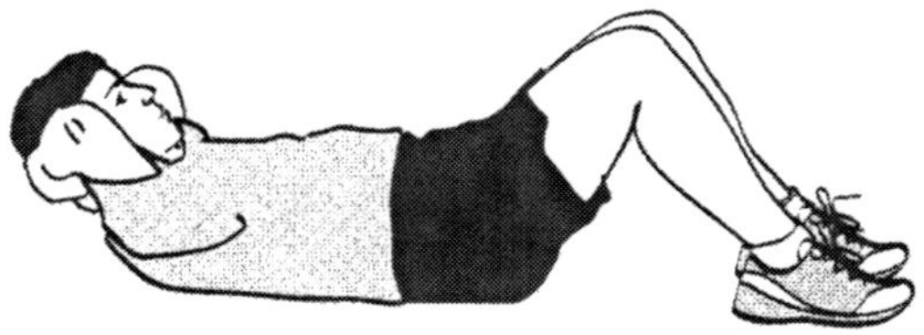

Crunches
Support the head and neck. Do three sets of 15.

Shoulders

The upper body has smaller muscle mass and therefore only 10 repetitions for each set of the following exercise are required. For the military press, strap your weights on your wrists using about 10 percent of your body weight on each one. If you prefer, you can also use hand weights or small barbells. With your elbows to the sides (not in front of you) and in line with your shoulders, lift your hands directly above your head and lower to the ears on each repetition. This exercise promotes the maintenance of the shoulder muscle groups.

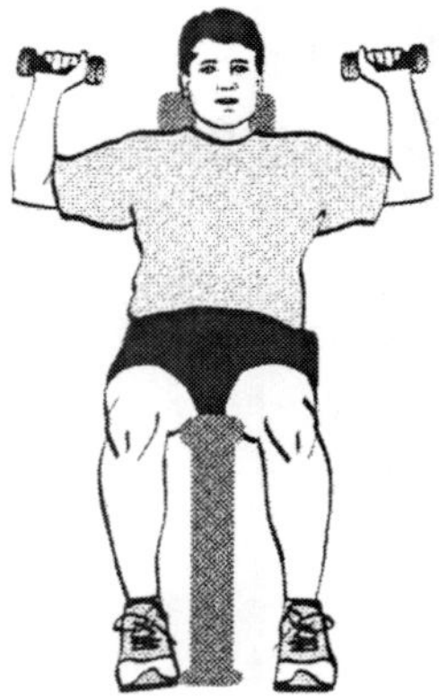

Military Press
Raise both arms above head. Do three sets of 10.

Pectorals I

The pectorals are the front chest muscles that you can exercise through resistance by pressing against the wall with both hands. Begin with arms straight and palms pressed against the wall. Lean into the wall and slowly bend your elbows until your chest touches the wall. Now push against the wall until your arms are straight again.

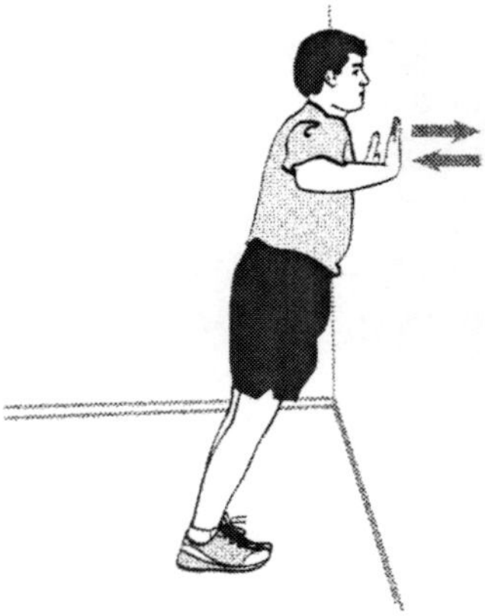

Chest Press
Push out with both arms. Do three sets of 10.

Pectorals II

After three sets of the chest press, the arms should be extended out to the sides and brought together to the middle of the body. Begin by raising your arms from your sides, in line with your shoulders, then bending the arms at a 90-degree angle. With your arms bent, rotate them to the front of your body, touching elbows, then rotate back sideways again. You should perform three sets of 10 for this routine.

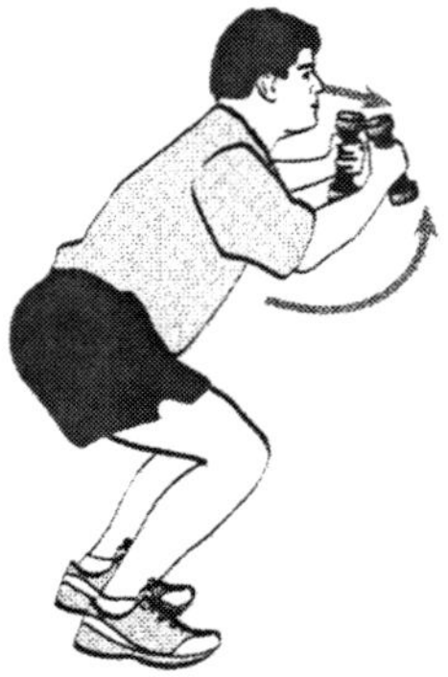

Pectoral Flys
Bring both arms to center of chest. Do three sets of 10.

Biceps

The biceps are located in the upper front of each arm and can be effectively exercised with hand or wrist weights. Extend both arms in front of your body with wrists up. Slowly curl your arm up toward your shoulder, then slowly extend. Do three sets of 10 repetitions on each arm.

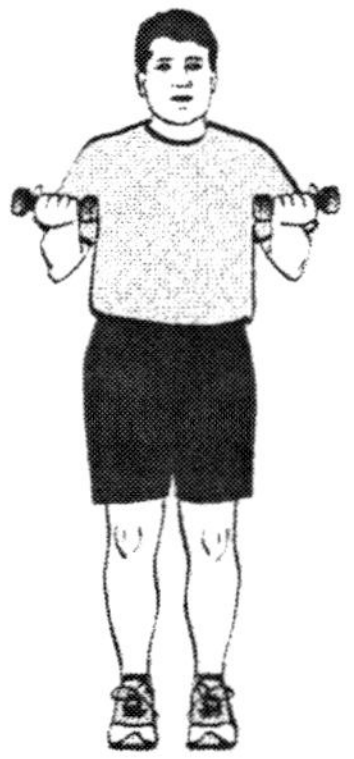

Biceps Curls
Curl up both arms. Do three sets of 10.

Triceps

The triceps are located at the back of each arm and can be effectively exercised by clasping your hands together over your head while holding hand weights or using wrist weights. Start with your arms extended over your head and hands together, then bend your arms at the elbow, touch the back of your head with your hands, and then extend your hands back to your starting position.

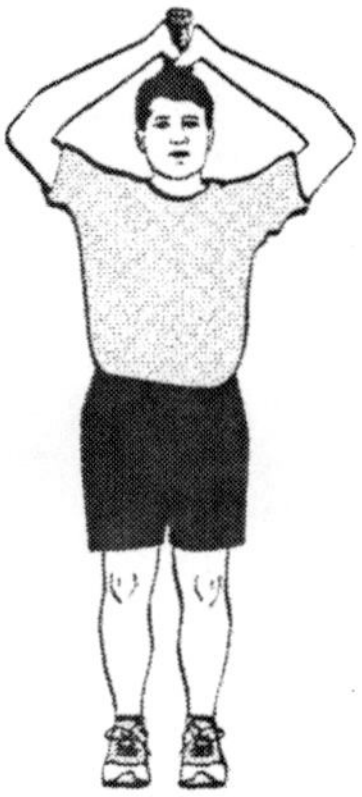

Triceps Curls
Both hands above head from shoulders and extend from back of shoulders. Do three sets of 10.

Key Points to Remember On Muscle Training

As the muscle mass is increased, weight can be increased to levels that are comfortable to suit individuals goals. (For beginners who are severely overweight the 15 percent and 10 percent for lower and upper body, respectively, might have to be reduced.) Additionally, make sure you keep moving while training with minimal pauses for taking small sips of water between each set. Hydration is critical to sound muscle training because it decreases soreness and promotes repair.

Exercises for the Endocrine Glands

Little attention, if any, is paid in the Western medical community to the health and maintenance of the endocrine glandular system. For the most part, the glands take care of themselves. It is generally believed that not much can be done to change their status other than using medications, supplements, or sometimes even surgery.

However, in the East, particularly in Tibet and some parts of northern India, exercises that promote glandular potency have been taught by Adepts for several thousand years. During the middle of the twentieth century these exercises were introduced to the West and they have proven to be helpful in maintaining and promoting balance between the seven endocrine glands. The glands known as the PPTTPAG group secrete important hormones into the bloodstream. The full names of these seven glands are the Pineal, Pituitary, Thyroid, Thymus, Pancreas, Adrenals, and the Gonads.

While Western medicine is only concerned with the mechanical workings of each of these glands, Eastern techniques focus on the invisible force vortex that spins clockwise around each gland. The vortex is actually part of the etheric body discussed in Chapter 5. Generally this vortex revolves at the same rate for each gland. Eastern Masters maintain that as long as this balanced rate of spin is equal, the glandular system is working properly and there is little chance of developing chronic health problems.

To maintain this balance, you can use the five endocrine exercises known as the Five Tibetan Rites. Each of these Tibetan Rites are described in the following sections and it is recommended they be performed daily to help ensure healthy maintenance of the glandular system.

With proper time and effort, most people can do the Five Tibetan Rites fairly easily to achieve the proper health benefits. If for some reason you are not able to do a particular rite as described, continue to do the ones that are comfortable for you. While performing the Tibetan Rites, breathe slowly, deeply, and evenly. There is a strong connection of benefits received to the quality of breathing while doing the rites. Oxygenated blood is vital for cell life and attention paid to maintaining a slow, deep breathing function will help ensure proper endocrine gland performance.

Tibetan Rite Number One Requires a Special Spin

Tibetan Rite number one does not resemble a typical yoga posture or exercise, but is a special spinning technique that helps to promote a synchronized internal movement of the vortices surrounding each endocrine gland. Of the five Tibetan Rites, this one is by far the most beneficial for keeping the vortices energized and is performed in the following way:

1. Stand erect with arms outstretched, horizontal to the floor, palms facing down. The arms, from the tip of the left hand to the tip of the right hand, should be in a near perfect straight line.
2. Turn from left to right, spinning around in a complete clockwise circle. Begin and end slowly, building up speed and slowing gradually. Breathe slowly and evenly as you spin.
3. Perform this rite for 21 full revolutions. Very few people can do all 21 revolutions the first time without getting seriously dizzy. Therefore, it is suggested that the student work up to 21 on a gradual basis in daily increments of adding three revolutions per day. At the end of seven days most will have no problem in performing 21 spins a day.

If at the end of seven days, you still feel dizziness, you might want to try a technique that dancers and ice skaters use to alleviate this problem. Focus your vision on a single point before you start spinning. As you turn, keep your eyes on that point as long as possible. When this point enters your vision again, refocus on it.

When you are finished spinning, relax your body by lying down and taking some deep breaths through your nose. Wait for any lingering dizziness to disappear. Do not begin the next rite until you feel completely balanced.

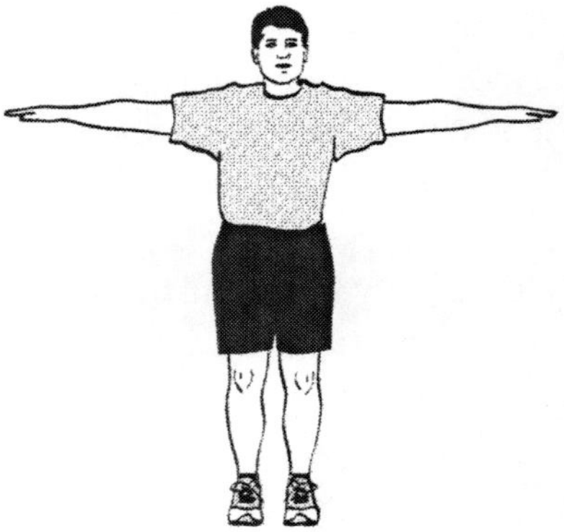

Tibetan Rite Number One
Turn clockwise with arms outstretched. Work up to 21 revolutions.

Tibetan Rite Number Two

Tibetan Rite number two has a special energy and massaging effect on the thyroid, adrenals, pancreas, kidneys, gonads, prostate, and the uterus. It's helpful in maintaining regular menstrual cycles and ameliorating the symptoms of menopause. It has a positive effect on the digestive system and it is good for promoting circulation, respiration, and toning the heart muscles.

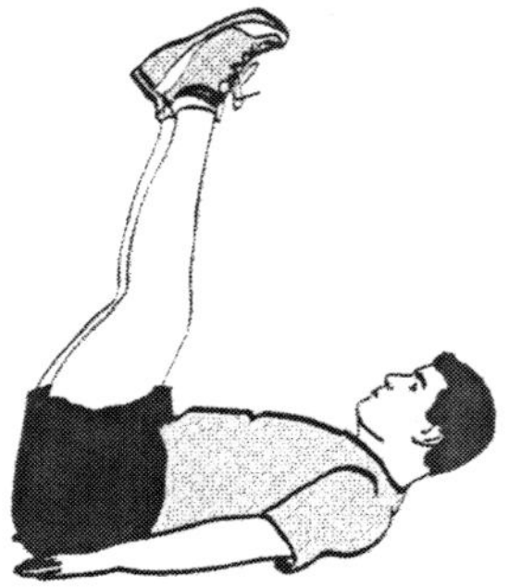

Tibetan Rite Number Two
Lie on floor and raise legs. Do 21 reps.

1. Lie flat on a mat or carpet, face up, legs extended. Place arms close to your sides, parallel to the body, palms down. (If you have a weak back, the hands can be placed under the upper gluteus maximus in order help support the lower back muscles.)
2. Breathe in through the nose as the head is raised off the floor, and tuck the chin against the chest. At the same time, lift both legs up, bringing them as close to vertical as possible. The straighter the legs can be kept, the more effective is the exercise on the glands and organs.
3. Slowly lower the head and the legs simultaneously, keeping the legs straight and breathing out through the nose.
4. Relax for a moment and then repeat the movement for a total of 21 repetitions. When starting out it is recommended that the repetitions be increased in increments of three a day until 21 can be accomplished over a seven-day period.

Tibetan Rite Number Three

Like Tibetan Rite number two, number three has similar beneficial effects on the thyroid, pancreas, adrenals, kidneys, gonads, prostate, and the uterus. Doing this movement will also increase your general sense of vitality and energy.

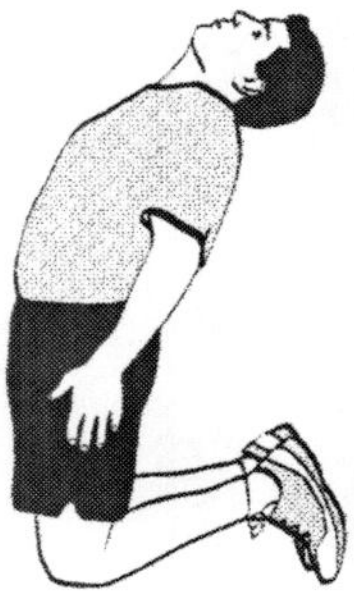

Tibetan Rite Number Three
Arch your back as you lean back. Do 21 reps.

1. Kneel on a carpet or mat, with your body in an erect position. Grasp the thighs with your thumbs facing forward, and breathe in through the nose.
2. Breathe out through the nose, as you gently roll the head and neck forward, tucking the chin against the chest.
3. Breathe in slowly and deeply as you lean backward, angling the torso over the lower legs. As the spine arches, bend the back gently as far as it can go.
4. Breathe out and return to the starting position. Breathe in and repeat the movement 21 times.

Very few have difficulty doing this exercise for 21 repetitions the first day, but if you are experiencing problems, work your way up in increments of three a day until you can do 21 repetitions.

Tibetan Rite Number Four

Tibetan Rite number four has a massaging and stimulating effect on the thyroid, thymus, adrenals, pancreas, and gonads. It also has an anaerobic muscle toning and fat burning impact over most of the body.

1. Sit on the floor, spine straight, legs fully extended in front, with feet apart about the width of the shoulders. Place palms down on the floor, alongside the buttocks with fingers pointing toward the toes and breathe in.

2. Breathe out and tuck the chin down against the chest. Breathe in again slowly as you let the head sink back as far as it will go. Raise the torso up as you continue with a slow, deep inhalation. The knees should be bent at a 90 degree angle over the feet, with the arms straight and perpendicular to the floor.

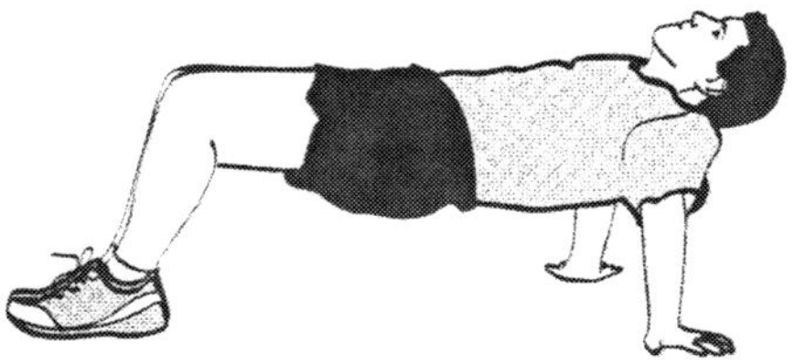

Tibetan Rite Number Four
Raise from a sitting position. Do 21 times.

3. In this position, tense every muscle in the body and hold your breath. Then breathe out slowly as every muscle is relaxed and return to the original position.
4. Rest a moment, breathe in, and repeat the movement for a total of 21 repetitions. If you experience difficulty, work your way up in increments of three a day until you can perform 21 repetitions.

Tibetan Rite Number Five

Tibetan Rite number five massages from a different angle and re-energizes all of the glands and organs affected in Tibetan Rite number four. It also has an anaerobic impact on fat burning and muscle maintenance throughout the body.

1. Start by lying face down with the legs extended and the toes curled under. The hands should be placed directly under the shoulders with the palms down. The feet should be spaced apart about the width of the shoulders, in line with the hands, forming a solid base.
2. Lift the body, including the legs, by fully extending the arms perpendicular to the floor and flexing the toes. This move resembles a modified push-up. The spine should be arched, the chest raised, and the lower back in a sagging position.

3. Slowly breathe in through the nose and gently move the head back as far as possible, push up with your toes and legs and bend the hips, bringing the body up into an inverted V. As you move into this position the head will naturally come forward. Tuck the chin against the chest so you can see the feet, which are now almost on the floor with only the heals slightly raised.
4. Breathe out as you return to the arched position with the arms and legs straight. Breathe in and repeat 21 times. If in the beginning doing 21 reps is too strenuous, use the incremental three-a-day increase over a seven-day period.

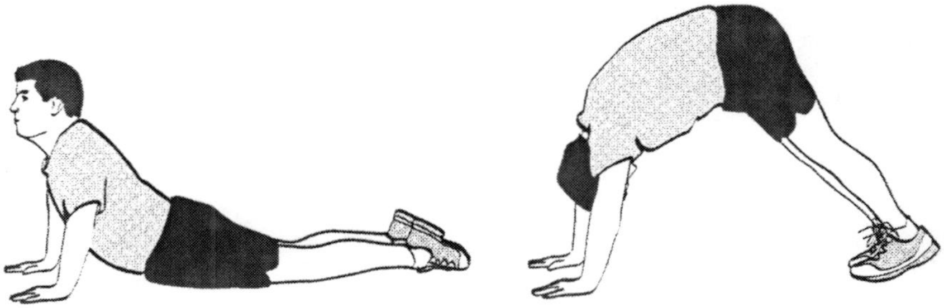

Tibetan Rite Number Five
Don't forget your breathing. Do 21 reps.

It may be helpful to spend five minutes or so relaxing after completing all five of the Tibetan Rites. This period should be one of deep, slow abdominal breathing, which will help release tension and stabilize the energy build-up impacting the endocrine glands and the surrounding vortexed chakras.

Benefits of the Five Tibetan Rites

Performing all five Tibetan Rites on a daily basis will likely have a significant impact on maintaining endocrine hormonal flow and balance, and will play a substantial role in wellness and longevity for your life. Performing the five Tibetan Rites takes on even more importance when consideration is given to all the increased opportunities for the exposure to toxins that are known to impede proper functioning of the glandular system. (For more information or more detailed descriptions of the five Tibetan Rites, look for *The Fountain of Youth* by Peter Kelder.)

Is All This Exercise Really Necessary?

Adhering to all of the components of the exercise principle may seem daunting in that it requires a commitment of about three hours a week. However, when looked at in conjunction with the other rules of wellness and longevity, an increase of many years of extended quality life can reasonably be expected to be added to the average life span as a result. Each person has to evaluate the worth of this result versus the effort required to achieve it. For some it is a no-brainer, but for others this quality life alternative may seem too difficult to realize. It's all a question of benefits and desires. Many case studies point to patients who have had a great deal of success with these techniques, even those who started in a state of denial. As mentioned in Chapters 1 and 2, if you want it, change can be easy and effective.

Dance to the Rhythm of the Soul

Getting one's body to follow the 7 Rite Rules of wellness, energy, and longevity can be viewed as a prescription for virtually ensuring membership in the centenarian club and further prepare you for fulfilling the prospect of immortality. The bottom line for making it happen comes from an inner willfulness, coupled with wisdom and active intelligence, for recognizing the benefits of adhering to rituals that can be intuitively sensed as being in sync with a rhythmic Soul.

To achieve this rhythm means overcoming the constant challenges presented by the desires of the emotional body. The emotional desires, if left unchecked, will eventually dominate the physical body and various addictive compulsive habits will likely occur. One of the proven processes for overcoming bad habits is to substitute with one or more of the exercise routines discussed in this chapter to aid in replacing a bad habit with a good habit.

CHAPTER 9

THE RITE RULE #7—SOULFULNESS

Control Your Body, Mind, and Emotions

Sometimes Jane would find herself sitting in her station wagon at a green light, the blare of horns jolting her out of a fog. Other times she would be putting away groceries, or taking a shower, or doing some other ordinary activity, when the tears would sneak up on her. Such was the grief that marked the days of this soft-spoken, 55-year-old legal secretary. And that was before her doctor diagnosed her with early stage breast cancer.

Her doctor's plan was to start Jane on chemotherapy, then radiation if the chemo didn't work, and if both methods failed, then surgery. One of Jane's friends at the law office urged her to come to me for a second opinion, and at our first consultation, Jane told me her story. "Two months after Tim, our son, started his freshman year at Ann Arbor, my husband announced he wanted a divorce. Not long after that, my mother died of a heart attack. All that within the last year and a half. And now this." Jane paused for a moment, then gave out a laugh. "If this weren't my real life, I'd say it was a badly written opera."

In addition to all the emotional stress, Jane was taxing her body by eating a diet that contained many toxins. She was also getting inadequate rest, water, and exercise. I knew that reclaiming a sense of physical and emotional well-being would give Jane the best chance of a positive outcome, and with her permission, I spoke to her doctor. He agreed to let Jane follow a four-week cleansing and lifestyle program of proper nutrition, rest, and exercise, along with my counseling, before starting her on chemotherapy.

After only four weeks of consciousness-raising therapy, coupled with following the 7 Rite Rules of energy, wellness, and longevity, Jane's medical tests showed her free of all cancer. Her doctor was in a state of disbelief. I wasn't surprised at all, just happy, happy that Jane had learned the 7 Rite Rules and was now living The Rite Way.

While Jane's outcome was uncommonly positive, someone in a less fortunate position would still see tremendous benefits from following my plan. The chemical and physical processes used by medical science today to treat invasive diseases like cancer are incredibly toxic—literally poisonous—but necessary in some cases to eradicate cancerous cells. Entering a treatment in less than optimum health—physically and emotionally—will reduce your chances for success. But living The Rite Way improves your health and reduces your risk for all of the chronic diseases listed in the matrix in the Introduction.

The "S" in the D-R-R-I-T-E-S acronym represents Soulfulness, which is the seventh rule of wellness and longevity. As with the other rules, this one directly contributes to enhancing your probability of achieving this physical immortality we've been discussing. The mind-body connection is a strong one, and employing the power of "belief" in this connection via a positive attitude is critical to maintaining the longevity of your physical body and achieving a rhythmic physical lifestyle.

Control of the body is the first step toward developing a connection with the Soul. But often, it's difficult to understand which comes first: gaining bodily control, or dealing effectively with emotional issues that can hamper physical progress. This dilemma deserves a great deal of attention because it's critical to your long-term success for health and wellness. The variables contributing to Soulfulness can go beyond the scope of the mind-body connection, and may have a great deal to do with your ability to control the emotional body. However, it's critically important since many studies support the position that the emotions are responsible for a significant number of chronic illnesses.

Is the Glass Half Full or Half Empty?

Characterization of attitude often employs the analogy as to whether a glass is perceived as half full or half empty. Depending on how you look at it, people often say that if you have a tendency to view the glass as half empty, you have a negative attitude. If you perceive the glass as half full, you generally view life's challenges with a positive attitude. Most people can easily relate to this generalization. Carrying this concept a little further, people with negative attitudes tend to make derogatory remarks and not be very supportive or constructive in difficult situations. Whereas someone with a positive attitude will most often make positive statements and be supportive and constructive in challenging situations. People with a positive attitude are perceived as demonstrating a genuine loving, caring, and harmless disposition toward all people with the overall intention of making the world a better place to live.

Impediments to a Positive Attitude

Research tells us that a negative attitude can promote feeling annoyed and stressed, whereas given the near identical situation, someone with a positive attitude shows no evidence of stress.

Conventional medicine holds the view that stress is the cause of many disorders and illnesses. However, when doctors examine disorders or symptoms brought on by stress, they often don't address the source of the stress. Even when some doctors do try to address the causes of stress, they look solely at external factors. In reality, all stress—no matter the external cause—is actually internally generated by one's level of consciousness. As the well-known quote says: "it is not life's events, but one's reaction to them that activates the symptoms of stress." A divorce can bring on agony or relief. Challenges on the job can result in positive stimulation or stress, depending on one's attitude. No matter what happens externally, stress is truly produced by one's own internal processing system.

Prevention Is Always Best

On the other hand, suggesting that one should simply think positively or change their perception may be easier said than done. If you're suffering from a chronic health problem, it can become a severe challenge to practice or maintain a positive attitude. For this reason alone it becomes very important to seriously follow the rules of wellness and longevity in order to prevent chronic disease. If one is suffering from chronic fatigue, asthma, arthritis, intestinal disorders, allergies, diabetes, ulcers, or obesity, one already has to overcome that hurdle of potential distraction. It's just one more impediment to developing and maintaining a positive attitude.

Negative Attitudes Can Have Physical Consequences

Even without the impediment of chronic disease, the destructive impact on the body from bouts of depression or anger can be serious and lead to chronic problems such as ulcers, headaches, digestive disorders, or hormonal imbalances. If you suffer from regular bouts of depression, you should seek professional help and be treated. The problem with negative thinking is that it can be so circular. Physical problems often serve as a precursor to negative thinking, and negative attitudes can lead to further physical disorders. The effects can be significant, not only adversely affecting the individual displaying the negative attitude, but also the people in contact with that individual.

From a purely individual and physiological standpoint, the choice you make about your attitude means your body is choosing between constructive anabolic endorphins and destructive catabolic adrenaline. To put it another way, you can create a sunny day internally or stir up a cell-damaging internal cyclone.

According to Dr. Hawkins in his book *Force Vs. Power*, the world of physics calls this internal cyclone "turbulence" and it is the subject of much research. When this turbulence occurs in the negative attractor fields of consciousness, it creates an emotional upset that continues until it establishes a new level of balance.

Dr. Hawkins believes when the mind is dominated by a negative world view, the direct result is a repetition of minute changes in energy flows to the various body organs. The subtle field of overall physiology is affected in all of its complex functions, mediated by electron transfer, neural hormonal balance, and nutritional status. Eventually, an accumulation of infinitesimal changes becomes discernible through measurement techniques such as electron microscopy, magnetic imaging or x-ray, or biochemical analysis. But by the time these changes are detectable, the dis-ease of negativity is already well advanced in its own self-perpetuating resonances.

Negative Attitudes Affect Physical Well-Being

The difference in negative attitude versus positive attitude and its effects on the body can clearly be shown through the use of Kirlian photography. Kirlian photography can measure the amount of aura or pranic energy emitted from the body. This photographic process can record a visual representation of spontaneous changes in the body as the body is subjected to stress. How does the process work? Simply stated, the subject being photographed is directed to think a negative thought. This puts stress on the body, and the aura surrounding the finger can be clearly seen as pushed away from the finger. The same person is then asked to think a positive thought, and this brings the aura back to the finger, indicating relief from the stress.

Other testing processes can show the effects of negative and/or positive thinking. Applied kinesiology, for example, is one of the most recently developed and most powerful processes available for measuring both negative and positive levels of consciousness.

Negative Thoughts Are Toxins to the Body

A negative attitude is a major toxin, equally as bad as any of the toxins mentioned in Chapter 7, negatively affecting the physical and the emotional body. A positive attitude, on the other hand, has been correlated to a number of good effects on the body including overcoming cancer, ulcers, digestion disorders, dementia, colds, headaches, and pre-menstrual syndrome.

Most of us intuitively know that a positive attitude will serve the body properly in the long run, but getting someone to recognize this truth when they are in the heat of a negative moment can be a major challenge. A great deal of the problem has to do with the formation of habits and how one has learned to view and deal with perceived negative conditions in their childhood years.

Much like the forming of addictive habits to food and or drink, negative attitudes, exhibited repeatedly, have a way of developing habit grooves in the subconscious. In order to pave over these grooves, one has to first recognize that a problem exists, and learn to believe in the conscious power of developing new grooves that will support a positive attitude and healthy lifestyle.

Belief in the Soul, Mind, Body, Emotion Connection

The concept of habit grooves in the subconscious can be expanded to include information-processing receptors present on every nerve cell membrane and probably present on most, if not all, of the body's cells. This finding was published by Candace Pert in her book *Molecules of Emotion*. Her remarkable experiments established that the "mind" is not only located the head but is distributed via signal molecules to the whole body. Her work emphasizes that emotions are not only derived through a feedback of the body's environmental information but that through sub- consciousness, the mind can use the brain to generate "molecules of emotion" and override the physical body. In other words, while proper use of conscious "belief" can bring health to an ill body, inappropriate sub-conscious control of emotions can easily make a healthy body diseased.

Belief in the power of energy that comes from your focused mind is clearly more potent than any chemical drug. This has been demonstrated in many studies and is particularly evident in the placebo effect, in which subjects have repeatedly shown that their belief that they are taking a drug trumps the effects of others who are actually relying on drugs. This syndrome is also evident with those who believe in hypnosis and the power of affirmations to overcome negative behaviors. When subjects believe in these therapies, the positive changes can be dramatic. To the extent that one believes the energy and power of the mind can connect and resonate with the Soul, as affirmed by many masters of wisdom, all things are possible, especially when combined with a consciousness of courage, acceptance, reason, and love.

Courage, Acceptance, Reason, and Love Are Levels of Consciousness that Contribute to Good Health

Your physical body knows when you are happy. Simply smiling can affect your attitude and others' reaction to you. Interjecting humor into your consciousness and conversations can have powerful positive impacts on your attitude and others when difficult and potentially stressful situations develop.

I like to compare the feelings generated from smiling and happiness to the image of a warm sunny day inside your body having therapeutic effects on all of your cells. If you consider this an ideal image and maintain it on a regular basis, it will underscore the importance of a positive attitude toward everything in life.

The wisdom of maintaining an accepting and loving attitude, as advocated by many Masters, including Jesus and Buddha, will have plenty of redeeming effects in everyday life. Simple observations will tell you that there is in fact an "accepting and loving" mindset connection to those who can maintain a positive attitude.

Shame, Guilt, Grief, and Anger Can Have Serious Negative Effects on Health

Negative emotions have been shown to contribute to a significant percentage of physical problems. If we use the analogy of destruction caused by tornadoes and hurricanes, you can imagine what may be happening within the human body when one exhibits intense anger.

Equally as damaging, depression can have a destructive impact on the body, leading to chronic problems such as ulcers, headaches, digestive disorders, and hormonal imbalances. Regular bouts of depression or anger need to be corrected. Seek professional help if these are re-occurring conditions.

As a holistic doctor, I recommend that a whole-body approach to treatment be applied with a focus on finding the primary cause or causes of the condition. In traditional approaches, diagnosis is made from primarily a symptomatic perspective.

Traditional doctors use pharmaceuticals such as Lithium, Prozac, Paxil, and others for treatment of depression. These drugs can lead to amelioration and/or suppression of symptoms, but by and large do not deal with the cause of the problem. Moreover, the side effects can be problematic. A diagnosis that does not take the whole person into account, and doesn't consider all of the 7 Rite Rules associated with lifestyles and their impact on the individual is, in my opinion, a potential disservice. In order to achieve long-term results that lead to overcoming the cause of depression, the health practitioner should have a thorough understanding of the patient's lifestyle habits as they relate to the 7 Rite Rules of wellness, energy, and longevity. An assessment of toxins and parasites, and testing for nutritional and hormonal imbalances and deficiencies should also be a part of the analysis.

Depression Could Be Caused by Poor Nutrition

Depression is a major impediment to achieving The Rite Soulfulness attitude for wellness and longevity. Negative levels of consciousness, including grief and depression, can sometimes be traced to nutritional deficiencies. Studies show that depression affects nearly 10 percent of the American population, roughly equal to 25 or 30 million people. This doesn't include the many people who function normally for the most part despite frequently finding themselves in low moods. Two-thirds of those who suffer from true depression are never treated and live their lives in misery without being recognized as victims of mental illness.

For the past 30 years psychiatry has been aware that certain bio-chemical changes in the brain can both influence and reflect changes in people's moods. A physical deficiency in any one of the chemicals responsible for maintaining good moods may lead to depression, just as a psychologically stressing factor in a person's life may manifest itself in the body by altering the sensitive chemical balance in the brain, thereby also causing depression or low moods. It the past 10 to 15 years specific brain chemicals called neurotransmitters have been isolated. These chemicals are released at the nerve endings in the brain and allow messages to be relayed throughout the rest of the brain and body.

A large number of depressed people have been found to have significant deficiencies in one or more of the neurotransmitters dopamine, norepinephrine, and serotonin. Dr. Null places these neurotransmitters in a chemical group called the amines, which are responsible for the control of emotions, sleep, pain, and many involuntary functions such as digestion.

Dr. Priscilla Slagle, a psychiatrist, states in her book *The Way Up from Down*, "Life style, age or genetics may cause a person to use up amines more rapidly than others." She points out that a defective receiving cell or re-uptake mechanism or a deficiency of the amino acids, vitamins, and minerals that make up amines could be the cause here. The nutrient deficiencies involved may result from excessive use of caffeine, sugar, alcohol, or tobacco. Sugar, coffee, alcohol, and tobacco all deplete and/or interfere with the formation of neurotransmitters by depleting B vitamins, vitamin C, zinc, magnesium, manganese, and tyrosine. These nutrients are all essential for maintaining a sense of well-being and good moods.

Toxins Can Be a Major Cause of Depression

In my own practice, I've helped a good number of patients with mood disorders by testing and correcting for nutrient deficiencies and toxic conditions. I've also helped a large number of people suffering from chronic depression through the use of parasite cleansing protocols. It appears that in some cases parasites, which I classify as a toxic condition, may be interfering with the brain's receptor sites for neurotransmitters. After parasite cleansing, patients report a dramatic reduction in mood disorders. (The parasite cleanse that I recommend is listed in the back of the book). Additional toxins, which could be interfering with the production of neurotransmitters and receptor sites, include metals such as mercury, lead, and aluminum. (Testing for these toxins can be performed by way of a hair analysis, and a laboratory kit available for that is also listed in the back of the book.)

Moreover, hair analysis, saliva, urine, and blood tests often reveal nutritional and amino acid deficiencies, which have been shown to be related to less than optimum neurotransmitter production. Simply supplementing some patients with amino acids such as tyrosine and tryptophan can work wonders in helping to stimulate the proper flow of the neurotransmitters serotonin and norepinephrine.

These options should serve to encourage those who may be suffering from mood disorders. A greater holistic understanding is underway helping identify many factors in mental illnesses caused by nutritional imbalances and toxic interferences. Each of these conditions is treatable and patients should make every effort to pursue natural ways for accomplishing treatment. I believe more attention should be given today to what kind of long-term effects many mood disorder prescription medications have on the body.

Setting Your Course for Controlling Body, Mind, and Emotions

As I discussed in Chapter 2, there are many processes and techniques for controlling your mind and moving negative attitudes into positive levels. If you can establish a rhythmic lifestyle, you can gain control of the physical body. Each of the 7 Rite Rules helps you achieve these goals. Even a small routine of exercising the body on a regular basis can stimulate the flow of the endorphin hormone, leading to optimizing the flow of the neurotransmitters and increasing positive feelings. Once you begin, you set up a cycle that helps you want to continue doing the exercises, which in turn helps promote a rhythmic lifestyle to foster the beginnings of a Soul connection.

What comes first to establish The Rite Soulfulness? Is it physical body control or emotional control? In my professional opinion, if you make a sincere attempt to follow the 7 Rite Rules you will in fact be establishing a bodily discipline and rhythm. This will serve you well in making the first step toward bodily control, which in turn will set up and enhance an initial connection with the Soul. You will likely find that in this process your emotional upheavals will be reduced and begin to ponder and contemplate further why and how you should employ some of the emotional control suggestions made in the body of this chapter. After all of this you will also began to realize that the mind has played a major role in gaining physical and emotional control, and will then begin to seek further ways to effectively control mental processes. The ability to control the body, emotions, and mental processes makes for a personality that can be qualified as having The Rite Soulfulness. In other words, you will be living The Rite Way and in accordance with the will of the Soul, which will of course help you prepare for immortality.

CHAPTER 10
LIVING THE RITE WAY
Well Worth the Effort

In the last nine chapters, I've given you the steps for embracing a lifelong wellness plan to increase your energy and longevity. If you take the 7 Rite Rules and reflect upon them, you'll find in place a sound foundation for all effort required. Their relative simplicity is such that it will be obvious that anyone who so chooses can live a vibrant, long-lived, disease-free life.

Prevention is a key component of The Rite Way, and I've tried to include extensive coverage on disease prevention with the expected payoff being a long life centered in wellness with increased energy. In theory, the 7 Rite Rules could substantially increase longevity and possibly prepare you for immortality. While everyone would agree that they would of course like to prevent all diseases, only a small percentage are actually willing to live the kind of lifestyles proven to be effective in this regard.

Why Won't Everyone Do It?

One is entitled to ask, "What is it about human nature that causes people to behave in ways that are detrimental to their long-term wellness and longevity?" For example, when some people are first exposed to the 7 Rite Rules of wellness, energy, and longevity, they tend to respond along the lines of "I'm going to enjoy life and I'm not going to be restricted by rules that will impair my satisfaction of food, drink, and a lifestyle that I find desirable on a daily basis." It's hard to recognize the cumulative effect of small actions on a day-to-day basis. And it's often only when the body starts to experience problems that we even know our bad behaviors have caught up with us.

Promoting Prevention Often Falls on Deaf Ears

The phrase "long term" is a key point when discussing chronic diseases. If a person doesn't get an immediate adverse reaction from a particular behavior, they are apt to assume little connection between the behavior and adverse long-term effects.

For example, a patient may be obese but often because of years of overeating marginal foods, they didn't connect the behavior with the adverse effects. Fat accumulation piles up slowly over months or years depending on the quantities and kinds of foods involved. The long-term effects are inevitable and obvious to most health-conscious people.

The Halo Effect, or It Won't Happen to Me

Other factors may account for this dissonance between proven health outcomes and negative behavior. The condition is generally referred to as the "halo effect," where individuals don't consider themselves to be part of that group at risk for heart disease, cancer, strokes, or diabetes. They perceive themselves and their conditions as different and therefore they are immune to the risks of smoking, overeating fast foods, sleep deprivation, dehydration, or sedentary habits. Some may say they are simply in denial or hooked. Many have become slaves to certain products or activities. Other health professionals could place them in a classification of pure ignorance. For whatever reason, they have not been able to connect the dots of negative behavior with patterns of chronic illnesses. A surprising number of people in this situation include otherwise bright and successful professionals with college degrees, living in the upper echelons of financial and social status. In some cases they maybe brilliant professors, businesspeople, financial experts, lawyers, or professionals able to give advice on how to prevent problems in their areas, but unable to change their personal lifestyle to prevent their own health problems.

It's Hard to Promote Prevention

Many institutions and health professionals give lip service to prevention of illnesses. Pharmaceutical corporations, health supplement companies, and most doctors get no monetary benefits from promoting prevention. In fact, if a national movement was started to raise the level of consciousness on wellness and other prevention lifestyles, health care as an industry would be alarmed. It takes an altruistic mindset of service—and a long-term view of the eventual better health effects—to effectively influence the general public in a meaningful way.

A Lifestyle of Disease Prevention Leads to Wellness, Energy, and Longevity

In view of all of the challenges surrounding the promotion of prevention, it will be clear to those who have implemented the 7 Rite Rules that disease prevention does in fact pay off far beyond the effort required to make it happen. I've repeated this concept many times and in different ways throughout the book, but even still some of my patients on occasion do not sufficiently grasp its significance. The principles are simple to remember:

- Living by the 7 Rite Rules will promote a lifestyle where the body's wisdom will insure the immune system as well as all other organs and systems to operate at optimum levels, virtually prohibiting illnesses. The prevention of virtually all diseases should be viewed as the foundation for experiencing a life full of wellness, energy, and longevity.
- If you have trouble sticking to the 7 Rite Rules due to compulsive habits or being in a state of denial, I urge you to actively seek help. If you take the time to review the material presented here, and apply it to your life, I believe you will be able to break bad habits and overcome the psychological and emotional roadblocks holding you back.

- The 7 Rite Rules are effective in preventing disease because they clearly show that eating nutritious solid foods, drinking pure liquids, and maintaining potent ordered energies are the key to helping the body wisdom work as designed.
- The ordered molecular energy inputs of sunlight, clean air, and etheric unseen ray energies are full of beneficial holistic and prevention effects. The internal processing of these energies in the form of proper rest, exercise, and their effect on emotions, mind, and body are clearly important.
- Living a toxin-free life is a critical piece to how all of these rules can be negated or adversely impacted with the toxic disordered energies that are so prevalent in animal products and man-made foods.

Those who have begun to implement the 7 Rite Rules will be feeling marked differences in their level of vitality. Over time they will clearly see increased levels of wellness with an absence of sickness, and in the long run it is likely that they will live a lot longer than most.

Words are cheap, but for those who have chosen to follow the words contained in the 7 Rite Rules of wellness, energy, and longevity, I am confident, due to my many experiences with hundreds of patients, that the elation that comes with increased vitality and the resulting absence of disease will be viewed as priceless.

Another Perspective on Why the Prospect of Immortality May Be Possible

While the possibility of physical body immortality may seem too absurd to even consider, I ask those who feel this way to review the fast-paced developments that are taking place in stem cell research, gene mapping, and organ replacements. There are many in the scientific medical field who claim that in 15 to 20 years, literally all body parts will be replaceable either through stem cell developments, DNA changes, or through surgeries. With these prospects in mind, the challenge to those who are resonating with the concepts presented in this work is to be there, with sound mind and body, when these exciting developments become practical.

Benefiting the Everlasting Soul May Supply Sufficient Motivation

And last but not least, to those who have little desire to stay in the same body for untold eons, the rationale for following the 7 Rite Rules in this lifetime offers the prospect for clearing all negative propensities while living The Rite Way to die healthy. When you can truly follow The Rite Way, making your body as healthy as possible, you may even help your Soul get an improved vehicle for the next go round.

Financial Health Insurance Benefits from Living THE RITE WAY

(updated information from insurance benefits stated in the introduction section)

Presently many billions of dollars are wasted on comprehensive health insurance premiums. It is common for employers to pay nearly $6,000 annually on comprehensive health insurance premiums. But now armed with the knowledge of Living the Rite Way you can approach your employer with an alternative high deductible Health Savings Account plan that could place $2500 annually into your Health Savings Account. Here's how it works:

Because you have agreed to accept a high deductible insurance that may cost less than $1,000 annually in premiums your employer may save $5,000 annually in premium payments. It will now be reasonable to suggest that $2500 per year be deposited in your Health Savings Account and your employer will net a savings of $2500 per year. A win win for both you and your employer because you can now use the Health Savings Account to fund all health expenses including the high deductible of possibly $1500 if a sickness requires extensive care. But now due to living The Rite Way your chances of sickness requiring extensive care are greatly reduced and your Health Savings Account will grow with compound interest at pre tax dollars. If you stay healthy over a 30 year period your Health Savings Account could be worth well over $100,000 with interest at retirement and the Account would be yours to spend as you like with Medicare now kicking in for your health insurance coverage.

If this concept holds an interest for you and your employer I would be pleased to advise as to the best way to implement such a plan for your benefit and maybe all employees in your company. E mail drrite@live.com

APPENDIX

Affirmations

The key to making the affirmation process effective is repetitive listening of all affirmations for at least 21 days. In addition, it might help to think of the process as one similar to programming a computer—the subconscious mind. It works best if you make positive present-tense statements. Whether you are presently living the way the affirmation states is not critical. What is important is that the affirmation get imprinted into your subconscious, as though you are performing the way it is stated, and over time you will feel a rhythm that will translate these subconscious imprints into bodily actions.

Following are general affirmations for weight loss and nutrition. Record these affirmations on tape and listen to them for 15 minutes in the morning and again for 15 minutes in the evening for 21 days. Use background music with a rhythm of approximately one beat per second. The background one-beat-per-second music increases the effectiveness of subconscious retention and is highly recommended. Read the affirmations slowly and in order, including the repetitive affirmations.

Talk to Yourself with The Rite Way Affirmations

1. I am a well-balanced, healthy, and happy person and love feeling good at all times.
2. I always eat the right amount of nutritious foods to keep me healthy.
3. My body is a temple where my soul resides and I do everything possible to treat my temple right and keep it in harmony with nature.
4. I always think positive thoughts.
5. I am a happy person because I feel good knowing I am healthy and in control of my emotions and eating habits.

6. I always eat the right portions of nutritious foods at mealtimes.
7. My blood pressure is just right because I keep a proper weight, exercise regularly, eat right, and always have a positive attitude.
8. I exercise regularly and always do the right things to keep me healthy.
9. I love life and enjoy being healthy.
10. My fat content is just right because I eat the right foods and exercise properly.
11. My triglyceride level is always OK because I always eat nutritious foods in the right amounts.
12. I love to help other people stay well and help them be happy.
13. My cholesterol level is just right because I love eating whole grains, fruits, vegetables, and other low-fat, wholesome foods.
14. I do all of the right things to keep my body in balance.
15. I always eat the right portions of nutritious foods at mealtimes.
16. My heart and lungs are in excellent condition because I get ample amounts of fresh air and sunshine, and of course exercise regularly.
17. My weight is just right because I love eating whole grains, fruits, vegetables, and other low-fat, wholesome foods.
18. My digestive system is in good order because I have a positive attitude and love feeling good naturally.
19. I love setting a good example, and living up to my responsibility of staying well.
20. My immune system is wonderful because I think positive thoughts, minimize stress, and eat and exercise properly.
21. Seeing myself as a healthy and confident person allows me to enjoy life and do my best.
22. My endocrine system is in balance and working perfectly because I eat right and do the prescribed endocrine exercises.
23. My mental attitude is just right because I follow good habits of proper rest and regular exposure to fresh air and sunshine.
24. I always eat the right portions of nutritious foods at mealtimes.
25. My emotions are always under control because I think right, behave right, eat right, and feel good all of the time.

26. I am committed to being a healthy person and I love knowing that my lifestyle will continue to keep me well with optimum longevity.
27. I always drink sufficient amounts of water during the day to ensure proper cleansing of my internal body.
28. I treat other people with respect and with their needs in mind, and care about their health, happiness, and well-being.
29. I always get sufficient amounts of rest, fresh air, and sunshine to ensure my immune system is maintained properly.
30. I have tremendous energy and enthusiasm all of the time.
31. I am highly motivated toward maintaining a healthy lifestyle.
32. Every situation is a positive learning experience for me.
33. I have health goals that I strive to meet on a daily basis.
34. I always eat the right portions of nutritious foods at mealtimes.
35. I always set a good example with love-motivated behavior.
36. Taking care of myself sets a good example and this supplies a worthwhile service to humanity.
37. Eating foods that are highly nutritious is energizing and allows me to accomplish everything I've set out to do.
38. Only I can control the way I feel and think, therefore I only feed my mind positive, healthy, and purposeful thoughts.
39. I always get sufficient rest and plenty of fresh air and sunshine, and enjoy being alive and feeling good.
40. I always listen to my body wisdom and its signals of comfort and discomfort.
41. I always live in the moment and have my attention on what is in front of me and see its fullness in every moment.
42. I always eat the right portions of nutritious foods at mealtimes.
43. I have total acceptance that this present moment is as it should be.
44. I regularly take time to be silent and meditate to calm the mind and body.
45. I really enjoy making this positive change in my life. It is exciting, energizing, satisfying, and fulfilling.
46. I love nutritious foods and living a toxin-free lifestyle.

47. I know and understand that the physical world mirrors my own consciousness; therefore I always think positive thoughts.
48. When I spend at least 30 minutes a day listening to my health affirmations I feel good and totally motivated to follow a healthy lifestyle.
49. I love living a healthy lifestyle where the right amount of exercise, rest, nutritious foods, water, fresh air, and sunshine are part of my everyday lifestyle.

Affirmations for Healthy Eating

1. I really enjoy eating natural raw foods.
2. I love eating fresh organic fruits, vegetables, raw nuts, seeds, and grains.
3. I enjoy the aroma of fresh, colorful fruits.
4. I receive a great deal of pleasure from just looking at fresh, colorful fruits and vegetables.
5. Knowing that the colors represent essential minerals heightens my enjoyment of all fruits and vegetables.
6. Eating raw nuts of almond and brazilian variety are especially nutritious.
7. The essential fatty acids, protein, and minerals contained in raw nuts make them very appealing to eat on a daily basis.
8. I love raw seeds; they provide balanced fresh oils and nutrition such as vitamins, minerals, proteins, and fiber.
9. I enjoy eating pumpkins, papaya, sunflower, and sesame seeds.
10. Green leafy vegetables are wonderfully filled with nutritious minerals and many anti-oxidants.
11. Green vegetables like wheat grass, broccoli, and peppers are extremely nutritious and are a part of all health-conscious diets.
12. A wide variety of fruits provides healthy nutrients and helps ensure proper enzyme and mineral intake.
13. Colorful deep purple and green grapes are delicious and wonderfully nutritious.
14. A large pink grapefruit tastes terrific and its ingredients help build strong immune systems.

15. I make sure that I eat 3 to 4 different fruits every day—they make perfect healthy snacks.
16. Large, firm, yellow bananas contain essential potassium that is known to help stabilize blood pressure.
17. Fresh carrots are filled with natural nutrients that literally help support good eyesight.
18. I love colorful green, yellow, and red fresh peppers. They have a great taste and furnish beneficial vitamins and minerals.
19. Dark green kale is an excellent source of calcium and I make it a part of every salad.
20. The colorful orange cantaloupe has a high density of vitamins and minerals, and I make a point to eat at least one per week.
21. Green and purple cabbage contain immense amounts of nutrients known to have anti-cancer properties.
22. Fresh watermelon has a special sweet taste and texture and is known to supply nutritious vitamins and minerals.
23. Raspberries have a very high biotin and fiber content and are very enjoyable with whole grains and other fruits like honeydew melons.
24. Soybean products like tofu and tempeh are examples of high-density, nutritious, clean protein.
25. Blue-green algae is excellent for ensuring that adequate amounts of vitamin B-12 are ingested.
26. All fruits and vegetables and most nuts and grains are desirable health-promoting foods.
27. Essential fatty acids such as those contained in flax, linseed, and hemp oils are nutritious when consumed on a daily basis.
28. Nuts like almonds are nutritious and alkaline forming and help support longevity.
29. I really enjoy eating raw natural foods.
30. Eating a fresh crunchy apple is one of the great joys of life.
31. The color, taste, and aroma of strawberries are truly magnificent.
32. When I eat a fresh, crunchy pear I know there is a great amount of nutrition being absorbed by my body.
33. Eating a large thick-skinned orange provides plenty bio-flavonoids and vitamin C.

34. A large bowl of red cherries presents a colorful and nutritious snack.
35. Fresh plums and peaches have a great taste and make me salivate just looking at them.
36. Fresh raw onions and garlic provide significant immune system building properties and are a part of every one of my dinners.
37. Flowering kale is one of the most nutritious leafy green vegetables, supplying plenty of calcium and protein with every bite.
38. Oatmeal and most vegetables help support the nervous system and mental balance by supplying vital amounts of vitamin B1.
39. Almonds, broccoli, and green leafy vegetables contain vitamin B2 and E that promotes healthy skin and good vision.
40. Legumes, bananas, and whole grains are filled with vitamin B3. These foods help prevent dermatitis, headaches, gum disease, and high blood pressure.
41. Brown rice, yams, whole grains, and broccoli contain large amounts of vitamin B5, a wonderful anti-oxidant that aids in the prevention of arthritis and high cholesterol.
42. Bananas, buckwheat, fish, avocados, and nuts are rich in vitamin B6, a major factor in red blood cell regeneration, and assists in the metabolism of amino acids and carbohydrates.
43. Citrus fruits, green peppers, tomatoes, and potatoes are rich in vitamin C, a primary factor in maintaining immune system strength.
44. I love eating fresh fruits, vegetables, and whole grains; they help increase my metabolism and naturally keep body fat at optimum levels.
45. I am so happy and satisfied to be on a healthy eating program of fresh fruits and vegetables, grains, nuts, and seeds. I'm feeling great and have plenty of energy, allowing me to enjoy life to its fullest.

LABORATORY TESTS

How to Measure Biological Age

Several of the most important biological markers are body composition, phase angle, skin elasticity, body balance, blood test heart markers, and history of illness. All tests unless otherwise stated should be performed by a doctor who has at least several years experience in analyzing all facets of the tests listed below (ask the doctor if he or she does these tests, and if so, how long have they been doing them):

- **Body composition** is determined with a bio-impedance device that electronically measures the amount of body fat on a percentage basis for the entire body. The optimum body fat for males is 15% and the optimum for females is 20%. Age 28 is considered as the standard starting point with the optimum fat percentages. Every percentage point of fat above the optimum adds two years to your biological age.
  Example: A male with a body fat of 30% is 15 percentage points above the optimum of 15% multiplied by two years for every point above the standard, and when added to 28 years would equate to a biological age of 58.
  (Bio-impedance devices can be found at most reputable health clubs, weight loss, and holistic health clinics.)
- **Phase angle** is also determined with a bio-impedance device and it supplies a number between 1 and 12 that equates to the amount of hydration within and outside the cells. The more water inside the cell, the higher the phase angle number. Using age 28 as the starting point, every point below 12 adds 5 years to biological age.
  Example: a phase angle of 6 would be multiplied by 5 for a total of 30 years added to 28, giving a biological age of 58.

- **Skin elasticity** is a bio-marker that most people can easily relate with in that it is primarily a visual test that can be performed without any tools as follows: Pinch about ½ inch of skin on the top of the left hand with the thumb and forefinger of the right hand. Hold the pinched skin for 5 seconds and after letting go, time the number of seconds required to get the skin back to level on the left hand. Add 10 years for every second required to get skin back to level.
  Example: 3 seconds would be multiplied by 10 for a total of 30 added to 28, giving a bio age of 58.
- **Body balance:** provides a bio-marker that combines the global functionality of the brain, muscles, and nerves with a simple balance test as follows: Lift the right foot 12 inches and extend it 12 inches in front while standing on the left foot. Both arms should be fully extended out horizontally from the sides. Note the time able to stay balanced (using a watch with a second hand). Do the test three times and average the amount of time able to stay balanced on one foot. Add % years for every second less than 21.
  Example: If the average balanced time is 17 seconds, multiply 4 times 5 years for a total of 20 years added to 28, giving a bio age of 48.
- **Cardiovascular assessment** analyzes blood for lipid markers, ratios, and independent risk factors. Together, these markers provide a thorough assessment of cardiovascular health status, revealing the biochemical environment associated with inflammation, lipid deposits, endothelial dysfunction, and clotting factors. The analyte markers measured include lipoprotein (a), homocysteine, fibrinogen, C-reactive protein, triglycerides, LDL & HDL cholesterol, apolipoprotein B, and apolipoprotein A1. The test requires 3ml of plasma, 4ml serum measured drawn locally, and the doctor will send samples to the Great Smokies Diagnostic Laboratory in North Carolina. The laboratory provides a color-coded risk assessment for each of the above analytes and a bio age is arrived at by adding 5 years for every marker in yellow and 10 years for every marker coded red.

Example: Homocysteine rated red=10 years, fibrinogen rated yellow=5 years, LDL rated red=10 years, C-reactive protein rated red=10 years for a total of 35 years added to the standard 28 years, giving a bio age of 63.

- **A history of illnesses** provides a bio-marker that measures the effectiveness of the immune system; it is determined by adding one year to the biological age for every illness encountered over the past three years (illness examples are those contained in the Illness Prevention Matrix displayed in the Introduction).
  Example: Every cold, flu, respiratory infection, or other illnesses encountered over the past three years adds one year to the biological age. If 5 illnesses were encountered over the past three years, add 5 years to the standard 28 (if the illness is chronic—like lupus or arthritis—add one year to the bio age for every year the disease existed).
- **Other bio-markers** include hearing, vision, blood pressure, and hand and body strength. These markers are only measured when the bio age exceeds a patient's calendar age on the first six markers.

BIBLIOGRAPHY

Atkins, R. *The New Diet Revolution*. New York: Avon Books, 1999.

Baily, A. *Esoteric Healing*. New York: Lucis Publishing Co., 1934.

Baily, A. *Esoteric Psychology*. New York: Lucis Publishing Co., 1938.

Beasley, J. *Betrayal of Health*. New York: Random House, Inc., 1992.

Becker, R. *The Body Electric*. New York: William Morrow & Co., 1985.

Batmanghelidj, F. *Your Body's Many Cries for Water*. Falls Church, Va.: Global Health Solutions, 1997.

Boritz, W. *Dare to be 100*. New York: Fireside, 1996.

Balvatsky, H. *The Secret Doctrine*. New York: Lucis Publishing, 1920.

Clark, H. *A Cure for All Diseases*. San Diego, Ca.: ProMotion Publishing, 1995.

Cousins, N. *Head First*. New York: Penguin Group, 1990.

Erasmus, U. *Fats That Heal, Fats That Kill*. Burnaby Canada, 1986.

Fossel, M. *Reversing Human Aging*. New York: William Morrow Inc., 1996.

Gerber, R. *Vibrational Medicine*. New York: Harper Collins, 2000.

Hawkins, D. *Power vs. Force*. Sedona, Arizona: Veritas Books, 2001.

Johnson, J. *The Path of the Masters*. Punjab, India. Radha Soami, 1939.

Kelder, M. *The Five Rites*. New York: Harcourt Brace, 1991.

Kurzweil, R. *Fantastic Voyage*. New York: Rodale, 2004.

Pert, C. *Molecules of Emotion*. New York: Scribner, 1997.

Pratt, G. *Instant Emotional Healing*. New York: Random House, 2000.

Prochaska, J. *Changing for Good*. New York: Avon Books, 1994.

Rampton, S. *Trust Us, We're Experts.* New York: Penguin Putman Inc., 2001.

Robins, J. *Diet for a New America.* Walpole, N.H.: Stillpoint Publishing, 1987.

Stitt, P. *Beating the Food Giants.* Manitowac, WI.: Natural Press, 1993.

Sui, C. *The Miracle of Pranic Healing.* Santa Monica, Ca.: Evergreen Publishing, 1999.

Yogananda, P. *Autobigraphy of a Yogi.* Los Angeles, Ca.: Self Realization Fellowship, 1946.

Index

B

D

O

P

Q

R

S

T

U

V

W

Additional Items Available from Dr. Rite

For additional information and products, visit Dr. Rite's website at http://www.theriteway.meta-ehealth.com.

Virtually every chronic disease is listed on this site with several research articles describing causes and remedies. Also many holistic products are listed and available for purchase.[1]

~

The following products referenced in *The Rite Way to Immortality* can be purchased directly from Dr. Rite:

- Weight loss and nutrition affirmations with appropriate background music (on cassette tape) are available for $20 plus $5 S&H.
- Testing kits for toxins and nearly all chronic health concerns (via saliva, urine, stool and blood samples) are available and can be obtained by e mailing dr.rite@centerforbetterhealth.com. You will be notified by e mail as to the cost and time of delivery. (If you are sure you have parasites and believe there is no need to perform a stool test, send $85.00 to the address below and 3 herbal remedies with instructions will be sent back ASAP).
- Arrangements to have your biological age measured can also be made by e-mailing dr.rite@centerforbetterhealth.com.

For all orders, send money or check payable to *Dr. Rite* to:

Dr. Rite
The Center for Better Health
1520 Nutmeg Pl.
Costa Mesa, CA 92626

1. Dr. Rite has a financial interest in the sale of these nutritional products.

Printed in the United States
150616LV00003B/118/P

9 781438 961934